# WHAT HAPPENED TO YOU?

## Also by
## Bruce D. Perry, M.D., Ph.D.

---

*The Boy Who Was Raised as a Dog: And Other Stories from a
Child Psychiatrist's Notebook (with Maia Szalavitz)*

*Brief: Reflections on Childhood, Trauma, and Society*

*Born for Love: Why Empathy Is Essential—and Endangered
(with Maia Szalavitz)*

## Also by Oprah Winfrey

---

*The Path Made Clear: Discovering Your Life's Direction
and Purpose*

*The Wisdom of Sundays: Life-Changing Insights from
Super Soul Conversations*

*Food, Health, and Happiness: 115 On-Point Recipes
for Great Meals and a Better Life*

*What I Know for Sure*

# WHAT HAPPENED TO YOU?

## CONVERSATIONS ON TRAUMA, RESILIENCE, AND HEALING

---

BRUCE D. PERRY, M.D., Ph.D.

OPRAH WINFREY

PUBLISHED BY

PRODUCED BY

FLATIRON
BOOKS
NEW YORK

MELCHER
MEDIA

In the discussions of Dr. Perry's clients, all names and many identifying details have been changed, and some discussions include a conflation of clinical situations.

www.flatironbooks.com

The Library of Congress Cataloging-in-Publication Data is available upon request.

ISBN 978-1-250-22318-0 (hardcover)
ISBN 978-1-250-22321-0 (ebook)

Our books may be purchased in bulk for promotional, educational, or business use. Please contact your local bookseller or the Macmillan Corporate and Premium Sales Department at 1-800-221-7945, extension 5442, or by email at MacmillanSpecialMarkets@macmillan.com.

First Edition: 2021

10 9 8 7 6 5 4 3 2 1

---

This book was produced by Melcher Media, Inc. / melcher.com
Interior design by Paul Kepple and Alex Bruce at Headcase Design
headcasedesign.com
Cover and interior illustrations by Henry Sene Yee
instagram.com/henryseneyee_draws/

# DEDICATION

---

BRUCE D. PERRY, M.D., PH.D.:

*For my clan:*
Barbara, Grant, Jay, Emily, Maddie, Benji, Elisabeth,
Katharine, Robert, and Emily

*In loving memory of*
Martha McGillis Perry

OPRAH WINFREY:

*To the daughter girls in my life who believed they had broken
wings. My hope for you is to not just fly but soar.*

# CONTENTS

# A Note from the Authors

This book is for anyone with a mother, father, partner, or child who may have experienced trauma. And, if you've ever had labels like "people pleaser," "self-sabotager," "disruptive," "argumentative," "checked out," "can't hold a job," or "bad at relationships" used to describe you or your loved ones, this book is for you. Or if you simply want to better understand yourself and others, this book is for you, too.

We know this reading experience will make you think and make you feel—and at times the feelings may be hard and painful. For some, the intense and sometimes disturbing content will be a challenge. For others, the concepts about the brain may be unfamiliar and initially difficult to understand. We ask for your patience and trust, with us and with yourselves.

When you find the reading too challenging, stop. Put the book down for an hour or a week. It will still be there when you feel able to return to it. And when you are ready to continue exploring why "what happened to you" shapes how you think, feel, and act, welcome. You just may discover a path forward.

# INTRODUCTION

---

*"Stop your crying," she would warn. "You better hush your mouth."*

*My face settled into stoic. My heart stopped racing. Biting hard into my lower lip so no words would escape me.*

*"I do this because I love you," she'd repeat her defense in my ear.*

*As a young girl, I was "whupped" regularly. At the time, it was accepted practice for caregivers to use corporal punishment to discipline a child. My grandmother, Hattie Mae, embraced it. But even at three years old, I knew that what I was experiencing was wrong.*

*One of the worst beatings I recall happened on a Sunday morning. Going to church played a major role in our lives. Just before we were to leave for service, I was sent to the well behind our house to pump water; the farmhouse where I lived with my grandparents did not have indoor plumbing. From the window, my grandmother caught a glimpse of me twirling my fingers in the water and became enraged. Though I was only daydreaming, innocently, as any child might, she was angry because this was our drinking water and I had put my fingers in it. She then asked me if I had been playing in the water and I said "no." She bent me over and whipped me so violently, my flesh welted. Afterward, I managed to put on my white Sunday-best dress; blood began to seep through and stain the crisp fabric a deep crimson. Livid at the sight, she chastised me for getting blood on my dress, then sent me to Sunday school. In the rural South, this is how black children were raised. There wasn't anyone I knew who wasn't whupped.*

*I was beaten for the slightest reasons. Spilled water, a broken glass, the inability to keep quiet or still. I heard a black comedian once say, "The longest walk is to get your own switch." I not only had to walk to get the switch, but, if there wasn't one available, I had to* go find one—a thin, young branch worked best, but if it was too thin I would have to braid two or three together to make it stronger. She often forced me to help her braid the switch. Sometimes the whuppings would get saved up for Saturday night when I was naked and freshly bathed.

Afterwards, when I could barely stand, she would tell me to "wipe that pout" off my face and start smiling. Bury it as though it never happened.

Eventually I developed a keen sense of when trouble was brewing. I recognized the shift in my grandmother's voice or the "look" that meant I had displeased her. She was not a mean person. I believe she cared for me and wanted me to be a "good girl." And I understood that "hushing my mouth" or silence was the only way to ensure a quick end to punishment and pain. For the next forty years, that pattern of conditioned compliance—the result of deeply rooted trauma—would define every relationship, interaction, and decision in my life.

The long-term impact of being whupped—then forced to hush and even smile about it—turned me into a world-class people pleaser for most of my life. It would not have taken me half a lifetime to learn to set boundaries and say "no" with confidence had I been nurtured differently.

As an adult, I am grateful to enjoy long-term, consistent, loving relationships with many people. Yet the early beatings, emotional fractures, and splintered connections that I experienced with the central figures in my early life no doubt helped develop my solitary independence. In the powerful words of the poem "Invictus," I am the captain of my soul and master of my fate.

Millions of people were treated just as I was as children and grew up believing their lives were of no value.

My conversations with Dr. Bruce Perry and the thousands of people who were brave enough to share their stories with me on The

Oprah Winfrey Show *have taught me that the effects of my treatment by those who were supposed to care for me weren't strictly emotional. There was also a biological response. Through my work with Dr. Perry, my eyes have been opened to the fact that although I experienced abuse and trauma as a child, my brain found ways to adapt.*

*This is where hope lives for all of us—in the unique adaptability of our miraculous brains. As Dr. Perry explains in this book, understanding how the brain reacts to stress or early trauma helps clarify how what has happened to us in the past shapes who we are, how we behave, and why we do the things we do.*

*Through this lens we can build a renewed sense of personal self-worth and ultimately recalibrate our responses to circumstances, situations, and relationships. It is, in other words, the key to reshaping our very lives.*

—Oprah Winfrey

One morning in 1989, I was sitting in my lab—the Laboratory of Developmental Neurosciences at the University of Chicago—looking at the results of a recent experiment, when my lab assistant poked his head into my office. "Oprah's calling you."

"Yeah, right. Take a message." I'd been up all night writing; the results of the experiment looked messed up. I wasn't in the mood for a practical joke.

He smirked. "No. Really. It's somebody from Harpo."

There was no possible reason for Oprah to call me. I was a young academic child psychiatrist studying the impact of stress and trauma on development. Only a handful of people knew about my work; most of my psychiatry peers didn't think much about the neurosciences or childhood trauma. The role of trauma as a major factor in physical and mental health was unexplored. I thought one of my friends was simply pranking me. But I took the call.

"Ms. Winfrey is convening a meeting of national leaders in the area of child abuse in Washington in two weeks. We would like you to attend."

After more explanation, it became clear that the meeting would be attended by many well-known and well-established people and organizations. My work—studying the impact of trauma on the developing brain—would be lost among more politically accepted, dominant perspectives. I politely declined.

Several weeks later, I received another call. "Oprah is inviting you to a daylong retreat at her farm in Indiana. There will be two other people, you, and Oprah. We want to brainstorm solutions to the issue of child abuse."

This time, with a chance to meaningfully contribute, I accepted.

The dominant voice that day was Andrew Vachss, an author and attorney specializing in representing children. His pioneering work highlighted the need to track known child abusers; at that point they could move from state to state, and there was no way to keep tabs on where they were or if they were complying with restrictions to avoid children. Our 1989 meeting in Indiana led to the 1991 drafting of the National Child Protection Act to establish a national database of convicted child abusers. On December 20, 1993, after two years of advocacy that included testifying before the U.S. Senate Judiciary Committee, the "Oprah Bill" was signed into law.

That day in 1989 led to many more conversations. Some took place on The Oprah Winfrey Show to discuss specific children's stories and campaigns on the importance of early childhood and brain development. Most of our conversations, however, were in the context of the Oprah Winfrey Leadership Academy for Girls (OWLAG), which Oprah founded in South Africa in 2007. This remarkable institution was created to select, support, educate, and enrich "disadvantaged" girls with high potential. The explicit intention was to create a cadre of future leaders. Many of these girls had demonstrated resilience and high academic achievement despite a range of adversities including poverty, traumatic loss, and community or intra-family violence. Early on, the school began to act on many of the concepts we discuss in this book; today, OWLAG is becoming a model of a trauma-sensitive, developmentally aware educational setting.

In 2018, I sat down with Oprah for a 60 Minutes story about "trauma-informed care." Though only two minutes of our conversation ended up in the final segment, millions of people were watching and listening, and the excitement created in the community of professionals working in trauma was remarkable. But there is so much more to say.

The enthusiasm for our conversation was in part a reflection of Oprah's own enthusiasm for the importance of this topic. On CBS This Morning, Oprah told Gayle King that she would dance on tabletops to get people to pay attention to the impact of trauma on the developing brains of children. In a CBS News supplement to the 60 Minutes show, Oprah called it the most important story of her life.

*Oprah has been talking about abuse, neglect, and healing for her entire career. Her dedication to educating people about trauma-related topics has been a hallmark of her shows. Millions of people have watched Oprah listen to, connect with, console, and learn from people with experience or expertise in trauma of all kinds. She has explored the impacts of traumatic loss, maltreatment, sexual abuse, racism, misogyny, domestic violence, community violence, gender and sexual identity issues, false imprisonment, and so much more, and through this has helped us explore health, healing, post-traumatic growth, and resilience.*

*For twenty-five years,* The Oprah Winfrey Show *took a deep and thoughtful look at developmental adversity, challenge, distress, stress, trauma, and resilience. She explored dissociative identity disorder in 1989; the importance of early-childhood experiences on brain development in 1997; the rights of adopted children in 2005; the impact of severe neglect in 2009; and much more. In many ways, her show paved the way for a larger, systemic awareness of these issues. Her final season included an episode featuring two hundred men, including Tyler Perry, disclosing their histories of sexual abuse. She has been and will continue to be a champion and guide for people impacted by adversity and trauma.*

*Oprah and I have been talking about trauma, the brain, resilience, and healing for more than thirty years, and this book is, in many ways, the culmination of those talks. It uses conversation and human stories to illuminate the science that underlies it all.*

*There are far too many aspects of development, the brain, and trauma to cover in one book, especially a book written through stories. The language and concepts used in this book translate the work of thousands of scientists, clinicians, and researchers in fields ranging from genetics to epidemiology to anthropology. It is a book for anyone and everyone.*

*The title* What Happened to You? *signifies a shift in perspective that honors the power of the past to shape our current functioning. The phrase originated in the pioneering work group of Dr. Sandra Bloom, developer of the Sanctuary Model. In Dr. Bloom's words:*

We [the treatment team for Sanctuary] were in a team meeting sometime around 1991 on our inpatient unit, trying to describe the change that had happened to us in recognizing and responding to the issue of trauma, especially what has become known now as childhood adversity—as a causal issue for the problems of most of the people we were treating—and Joe Foderaro, LCSW, always good at pithy observations, said, "It's that we have changed our fundamental question from 'What's wrong with you?' to 'What happened to you?'"

*Oprah and I are convinced that asking the fundamental question "What happened to you?" can help each of us know a little more about how experiences—both good and bad—shape us. Our hope in sharing these stories and scientific concepts is that every reader will, in their own way, gain insights to help us all live better, more fulfilling lives.*

—Dr. Bruce Perry

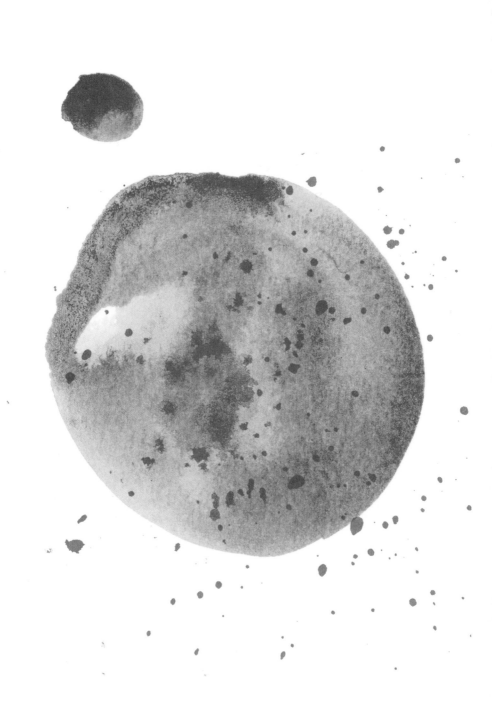

# CHAPTER 1

———

# MAKING SENSE OF THE WORLD

*More than 130 million babies are born in the world every year. Each arrives into their own unique set of social, economic, and cultural circumstances. Some are welcomed with gratitude and joy, cradled in the arms of their ecstatic parents and family. Others are more like me, experiencing rejection from a young mother who dreamed of a different life, a couple crushed by the pressures of poverty, an enraged father perpetuating a cycle of abuse.*

*Yet whether or not they're loved, every current and former newborn (that's you and me) shares one profoundly important trait. Despite the myriad circumstances into which we're born, we come into the world with an innate sense of wholeness. We don't begin our lives by asking: Am I enough? Am I worthy? Am I deserving or lovable?*

*Not one baby in the earliest moments of awareness asks, "Do I matter?" Their world is a place of wonder. But with their very first breaths, these tiny human beings begin trying to make sense of their surroundings. Who will nurture and care for them? What will bring comfort? And for so many little ones, life begins to take its toll, with violent eruptions by the caregiver or simply the lack of a soothing voice or a gentle touch. In our first encounters, our human experiences diverge.*

*The most pervasive feeling I remember from my own childhood is loneliness. My mother and father were together only once, underneath an old oak tree not far from the house where my mother, Vernita, was raised in Kosciusko, Mississippi. My father, Vernon, used to tell me I would never have been born if he hadn't been curious about what was underneath my mother's pink poodle skirt. Nine months after that singular encounter, I arrived. From the moment I could make sense of it, I knew I was unwanted. My father didn't even know about me until my mother sent him a birth announcement and asked for money to buy baby clothes.*

*My grandmother Hattie Mae's home was a place where children were seen and not heard. I have distinct memories of my grandfather shooing me away with his cane—yet no memory of him speaking directly to me. After my grandmother passed away, I was shuttled between my mother, who had moved to Milwaukee, and my father, in Nashville. Because I didn't know either one, I struggled to develop strong roots or connections with my parents. My mother worked as a maid for fifty dollars a week in Fox Point, on the North Shore of Milwaukee, doing what she could to care for three young children. There was no time for nurturing. I was always trying not to bother her or worry her. My mother felt distant, cold to the needs of this little girl. All of the energy went to keeping her head above water, surviving. I always felt like a burden, an "extra mouth to feed." I rarely remember feeling loved. From as early as I can remember, I knew I was on my own.*

*What I've learned from talking to so many victims of traumatic events, abuse, or neglect is that after absorbing these painful experiences, the child begins to ache. A deep longing to feel needed, validated, and valued begins to take hold. As these children grow, they lack the ability to set a standard for what they deserve. And if that lack is not addressed, what often follows is a complicated, frustrating pattern of self-sabotage, violence, promiscuity, or addiction.*

*This is where the work begins—the work to excavate the roots that were put down long before we had the words to articulate what was happening to us.*

*Dr. Perry has helped open my eyes to the ways in which powerful, frightening, or isolating sensory experiences that last mere seconds or are endured for years can remain locked deep in the brain. Yet as our brains develop, constantly absorbing new experiences while continuing to make sense of the world around us, every moment builds upon all the moments that came before.*

*I have always felt the truth of the saying that the acorn contains the oak. And through my work with Dr. Perry, I know this to be true, too: If we want to understand the oak, it's back to the acorn we must go.*

—Oprah

*Early in our relationship, I remember Oprah saying, "You're the guy who sees everything through the lens of the brain. Do you think about the brain all the time?" The short answer is,* almost. *I think about the brain a lot. I was trained as a neuroscientist and have been studying the brain and stress-response systems since I was in college. I'm also a psychiatrist, a field I pursued after my training in the neurosciences. I've found that a "brain-aware" perspective helps me when I'm trying to understand people.*

*Being a child psychiatrist, I'm often asked about troubling behaviors. Why is that child acting like a baby? Can't he act his age? How could a mother stand by and watch her boyfriend beat her child? Why would someone ever abuse a child? What is wrong with that child? That mother? That boyfriend?*

*Over the years, I've found that seemingly senseless behavior makes sense once you look at what is behind it. And since the brain is the part of us that allows us to think, feel, and act, whenever I'm trying to understand someone, I wonder about that person's brain.* Why did they do that? What would make them act that way? *Something happened that influenced how their brain works.*

*The first time I was able to use this neuroscience lens to understand behavior, I was a young psychiatrist, still training. I was working with an elderly man, Mike Roseman—a smart, funny, kind man. Mike was a veteran of the Korean War and had seen lots of combat. He had classic PTSD (post-traumatic stress disorder) symptoms, which we'll talk about in a deeper way later; he suffered with anxiety, sleep difficulties, depression, and episodic flashbacks in which he literally felt as if he was in combat. He had resorted to self-medicating with alcohol and struggled with binge drinking. This, of course, contributed to work and family conflicts, and ultimately led to divorce and forced retirement.*

*We had been working together for about a year, and Mike had been doing pretty well managing his drinking, but his other symptoms persisted.*

*One day he called, very upset. "Doc, can I come in and see you today? It's important. And Sally wants to come." Sally was a retired* teacher Mike had been dating; he'd talked a lot in previous sessions about not wanting to "blow this one." Sensing the urgency, I agreed.

Later that afternoon, they came into my office and sat next to each other on the couch. They were holding hands. Sally gently whispered in his ear; Mike looked shamed, and it was clear she was trying to reassure him. They looked like nervous teenagers.

He started. "Can you explain PTSD to her? You know, why I'm all messed up." He started to tear up. "What's wrong with me? Korea was over thirty years ago." Sally moved to hold him.

I felt myself floundering—could I really explain PTSD?—so I stalled. "If I may ask: Why now, Mike? Did something happen?"

"We were going out last night. Had a nice dinner and we were walking downtown on our way to the movies. And suddenly I was in the street, between parked cars, on my belly with my hands over my head, terrified. I thought we were being shot at. I was pretty confused, I guess. At some point, I realized that a motorcycle had backfired. Sounded like gunfire. The knees on my suit were torn. I was sweaty, my heart was racing. I was so embarrassed. Felt like I was jumping out of my skin. I just wanted to go home and get drunk."

Sally said, "One minute we were arm in arm, the next he is back in a foxhole in Korea, screaming. I tried to get down and help him, but he just pushed me away. He hit me." She paused. "It seems like it lasted for ten minutes, but I think it was only a couple of minutes. Tell me how to help him." She turned to look at Mike. "I'm not giving up on you."

"Tell her what's wrong with me," he pleaded.

This was 1985. Research on PTSD was still very preliminary, and I was a twenty-nine-year-old inexperienced psychiatrist-in-training; I didn't know squat. "Listen, I don't know if I have any answers here," I said. "But I do know that Mike was not trying to hurt you."

"I know that." Sally looked at me like I was an idiot—the idiot I actually was. But while I didn't know much about clinical work, I did know a lot about the brain, memory, and the stress response. I thought about Mike jumping for cover in the street, not as a clinician but as a neuroscientist. What was going on in his brain when that motorcycle backfired? I started to look at a clinical problem through the lens of the brain.

"I think part of the problem is that many years ago, in Korea, Mike's brain adapted to continuous threat—his body and brain became oversensitive and overreactive to any threat-related signals from the world. Back then, to stay alive, his brain made a connection—basically a specialized form of memory—between the sounds of gunfire and shelling and the need to activate an extreme survival response." I paused. "Does that make sense?"

Sally nodded. "He is jumpy."

"Mike, I've seen you flinch and startle in my office many times when a door slams or a cart rattles too loud in the hallway. You're always scanning the room, too. Any little shift in activity, sound, light draws your attention."

"If you didn't keep your head down," Mike said, "you were dead. If you weren't vigilant at night, you were dead. If you fell asleep, you were dead." He stared into space, unblinking. After a moment of silence, he sighed. "I hate the Fourth of July. And New Year's. The fireworks make me jump out of my skin. Even if I know there will be fireworks, I still jump—my heart feels like it will burst out of my chest. I hate it. I can't sleep for a week after that."

"Right. So that original adaptive and protective memory is still there. It hasn't gone away."

"But he doesn't need it anymore," Sally said. "It's actually making his life miserable. Can't he just unlearn it?"

"That is a great question," I said. "The tricky part is that not all of these combat-related memories are in parts of the brain Mike can consciously control. Let me try to explain this a bit."

I pulled out a piece of paper and drew an upside-down triangle and three lines dividing it into four parts. It was the first time I'd represented the brain that way. Thirty-five years later, we still use this basic model to help teach about the brain, stress, and trauma.

"Let's look at the basic organization of the brain. It's like a four-layered cake. At the top is the cortex, the most uniquely human part of our brain." I started labeling my drawing with different brain-mediated functions, as in the illustration, opposite.

As I did, I explained: "The systems at the top are responsible for speech and language, thinking, planning; our values and beliefs are stored there. And, very important for you, this is the part of the brain that can 'tell time.' When the cortex is 'online' and active, we can think about the past and look forward to the future. We know which things are in our past and which things are present, yes?" Mike and Sally nodded.

"Okay. Now look at the bottom of the brain—the brainstem. This part of the brain controls less complex, mostly regulatory, functions like body-temperature regulation, breathing, heart rate, and so forth. But there are no networks in the bottom part that think or tell time. Sometimes we refer to this part of the brain as the reptilian brain, so think of what a lizard can do—they don't plan much, or think; they mostly live in the moment and react. But we humans, thanks to the top part of our brain—the cortex—can invent, create, plan, and tell time."

I looked at them to make sure they were tracking with me before continuing.

"Input from all of our senses—vision, hearing, touch, smell—first comes into our brain in the lower areas. None of our sensory input goes directly to the cortex; everything first connects to lower parts of the brain."

They nodded.

"Once the signal comes into the brainstem"—here I directed their attention to the bottom of the triangle—"it is processed. Basically, the incoming signal is matched against previously stored experiences. In this case, the matching process connected the motorcycle backfire with gunfire—remember that combat-related memory? And since

# Figure 1

## A MODEL OF THE BRAIN

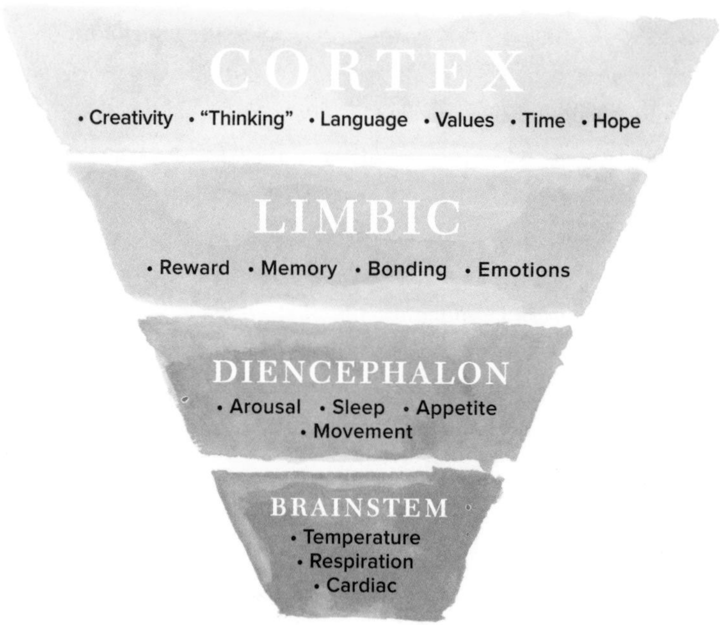

**CORTEX**
- Creativity  - "Thinking"  - Language  - Values  - Time  - Hope

**LIMBIC**
- Reward  - Memory  - Bonding  - Emotions

**DIENCEPHALON**
- Arousal  - Sleep  - Appetite
- Movement

**BRAINSTEM**
- Temperature
- Respiration
- Cardiac

HIERARCHICAL ORGANIZATION OF THE HUMAN BRAIN

The brain can be divided into four interconnected areas: brainstem, diencephalon, limbic, and cortex. The structural and functional complexity increases from the lower, simpler areas of the brainstem up to the cortex. The cortex mediates the most uniquely "human" functions such as speech and language, abstract cognition, and the capacity to reflect on the past and envision the future.

*your brainstem can't tell time, or know that many years have passed, it activates the stress response and you have a full-blown threat response. You feel and act as if you are under attack. Your brainstem can't say, 'Hey, don't get so stirred up, Korea was thirty years ago. That sound was simply a motorcycle backfiring.'"*

*I watched this sink in. "Now, when the signal finally gets up to the cortex, the cortex can figure out what's really going on. But one of the first things that happens when you activate the stress response is that systems in the higher parts of the brain, including our ability to 'tell time,' get shut down. So the information about the motorcycle backfire did ultimately get to the cortex, but it took a while. And until it did, you were back in Korea and then confused. It took you all night to calm down, right?"*

*"I didn't sleep at all." Mike looked exhausted but relieved. "So I'm not crazy?"*

*"No. Your brain is doing exactly what you would expect it to do considering what you lived through. But what was once adaptive has become maladaptive. What kept you alive in Korea is killing you back home. We have to figure out how to help your stress-response systems become less reactive and supersensitive."*

*That, of course, is not the end of Mike's story, but the understanding of what was "underneath" his confusing behavior was very comforting for him and Sally. For me, it started a much more active process of integrating principles from the neurosciences into clinical practice. It illuminated how "evocative cues"—basically any sensory input, like a sight, sound, smell, taste, or touch—can activate a traumatic memory. In Mike's case, the motorcycle backfire evoked the complex memory of combat. And it was one of the first examples I shared with Oprah when we began to discuss trauma.*

*Oprah*: When I hear Mr. Roseman's story, the first thing I notice is that he felt flawed; he even asks, "What is wrong with me?" But you focused on "What happened to me?" rather than "What's wrong with me?"—which is exactly the shift we're trying to help others make.

His story also helped me really understand what you mean when you talk about the "sequential" organization of the brain.

*Dr. Perry*: All experience is processed from the bottom up, meaning, to get to the top, "smart" part of our brain, we have to go through the lower, not-so-smart part. This sequential processing means that the most primitive, reactive part of our brain is the first part to interpret and act on the information coming in from our senses. Bottom line: *Our brain is organized to act and feel before we think.* This is also how our brain develops—sequentially, from the bottom up. The developing infant *acts* and *feels,* and these actions and feelings help organize how they will begin to *think.*

*Oprah*: For years, you've been telling me that the earliest experiences have the biggest impact because that is when the brain is most rapidly growing.

*Dr. Perry*: Not only is "What happened to you?" the key question if you want to understand someone, it is the key question if you want to understand the brain. In other words, your personal history—the people and places in your life—influences your brain's development. The result is that each of our brains is unique. Our life experiences shape the way key systems in our brain organize and function. So each of us sees and understands the world in a unique way.

The example of Mr. Roseman involves traumatic experiences that took place when he was twenty-four years old. If these experiences changed the brain of a twenty-four-year-old, imagine the impact of trauma on the brain of an infant or toddler—how much more pervasive the effects would be.

Starting in the womb, the developing brain begins to store parts of our life experience. Fetal brain development can be influenced by a host of factors including mother's stress; drug, alcohol, and nicotine intake; diet; and patterns of activity. During the first nine months, development is explosive, at times reaching a rate of twenty thousand new neurons "born" each second. (In comparison, an adult may, on a good day, create seven hundred new neurons.) By birth, the new-born has 86 billion neurons; these will continue to grow and connect to create complex networks that allow the newborn to begin making sense of their world. This is all extremely complex and not fully understood by researchers, but there are a few basic principles that will be helpful throughout our conversations about how this relates to trauma.

Our external senses—sight, sound, smell, taste, and touch—monitor what is going on outside of our body. To do this, they rely on the sensory organs—eyes, ears, nose, and skin. When these are stimulated by light, sound, smell, or touch, specialized neurons send a signal into the brain.

We also have sensory systems that tell us what is going on inside our body. This is called interoception, and it creates our sense of, for instance, being thirsty, hungry, or short of breath. All the sensory inputs from the outside world and our inside world give continuous feedback to the brain so that the proper systems can be activated to keep us healthy and safe. If we're thirsty, we seek water; if we're hungry, we seek food; if we sense danger, we mobilize our stress-response systems.

The brain categorizes every bit of sensory input and sends it "up the triangle" to other parts of the brain to integrate and process it further. This creates an increasingly rich and detailed version of any experience, as various inputs become linked based on how they're sorted. For example, the brain sends some visual input to the same areas it sends auditory (sound), tactile (touch), and olfactory (smell) sensations that come in at exactly the same time. These different sensations—the sights, sounds, smells, and movements of the same experience—then become connected. This is the beginning of making sense of the world.

As your brain starts to create the complex memories that store these connections, your personal catalog of experiences is being created. As we grow up, we are all trying to make sense of what's happening around us. What does that sound mean? What does it mean when someone rubs my back? What does that expression on his face mean? What else happens when that scent is present?

For one child, eye contact means, "I care for you; I'm interested in you." For another it may mean, "I'm about to yell at you." Moment by moment in early life, our developing brain sorts and stores our personal experiences, making our personal "codebook" that helps us interpret the world. Each of us creates a unique worldview shaped by our life's experiences.

Imagine, for a moment, the dramatic changes in the sensory world of a newborn. Their world, once warm, rhythmic, and dark, becomes, at the moment of birth, an overwhelming sensory bath of images, sounds, temperature shifts, and exposure to air. The brain is bombarded by new patterns of sensory input. And because so much of the world is new when you're a baby, that's when your brain is most rapidly and actively making these new connections. The experiences in the first years of life are disproportionately powerful in shaping how your brain organizes.

Oprah: One of the most important things I've learned from your research is that young children absorb so much more than we realize. The younger you are, the more sensitive you are to your emotional climate. People feel like they can curse in front of young children. They believe they can be violent in front of young children. I've done hundreds of shows where mothers said, "Well, when he gets older, I'll leave the abusive father"—thinking, *My child's too young to understand,* when, in fact, it's exactly the opposite.

*Dr. Perry*: Yes, it's exactly the opposite. The younger you are, the more you depend upon your caregivers—parents and other adults—to help you interpret the world. In some ways, the young child experiences the world through the filters of these adults.

While a very young child may not understand the words used in language, they do sense the nonverbal parts of communication, like tone of voice. They can feel the tension and hostility in angry speech, and the exhaustion and despair of depressed language. And because the brain is growing so rapidly in the first years of life and creating thousands upon thousands of associations about how the world works, these early experiences have more impact on the infant and young child.

For example, when children have abusive fathers, their brains begin to connect men with threat, anger, and fear. And this worldview gets built in—men are dangerous, threatening, they will hurt you and the people you love. If that is your ingrained view of the world, imagine what happens when you have a male teacher or coach. Imagine how you will view a new, healthy, non-abusive man in your mother's life.

*Oprah*: And when you haven't developed the words or ability to identify what you see or feel, you're just operating on vibration. And the vibration in the house is . . . *this is bad.*

*Dr. Perry*: That vibration, as you describe it, equates to the emotional tone of the environment.

*Oprah*: Yes, I believe every environment has a tone. If you were to walk into any home as a stranger, not speaking the language, you could absolutely feel whether this is a place where people are loved. Just as you can sense when something's off. You may not know what it is, but something feels off.

*Dr. Perry*: And in the same way, you could walk into a preschool and say, "Wow, this is a great environment." You can feel the climate, the emotional tone. And you could go to a different classroom in the same school and say, "Whoa, what's going on here?" It's so powerful. There are parts of our brain that are very, very sensitive to nonverbal relational cues. And in our society, this is an underappreciated aspect of the way human beings work. We tend to be a very verbal society—written and spoken words are important—but the majority of communication is actually nonverbal.

*Oprah*: You teach that when you experience trauma in the first years of life, meaning from birth through age two—before you've developed the ability to explain the event—it can have a deeper impact on your brain than when you actually do have the words to explain it.

I think about children who are molested when they are so young that they don't have the language to process what has happened. The experience locks into the brain in a way it wouldn't if the child could express with words what happened.

*Dr. Perry*: What you're describing here is a form of memory. Let's turn back to the upside-down triangle I drew for Mr. Roseman.

Each biological system in our body has some way to change in response to experience; in a sense, then, that change is a record of past experiences—or, basically, memory. Neurons are exquisitely sensitive to experience, and neural networks in every part of the brain can make memory. Remembering names, phone numbers, and where you left your keys is a function of the neural networks of the cortex. But we also have emotional memories: A song can elicit a feeling, an association with an experience that took place years ago. The smell of roasted turkey or freshly baked bread may elicit a warm sense of belonging, or a melancholy sense of a lost past. These feelings arise from associations stored in the neural networks of the limbic and other brain regions. And there are motor-vestibular memories—curling up in the fetal position is essentially an act of remembering—stored in even lower networks in the brain. But traumatic experience can create complex memory traces that involve *all* regions of the brain.

As we've mentioned already, the brain develops sequentially, from the bottom up and the inside out, from the basic functions of the brainstem to the complex achievements of the cortex. Each brain area has the capacity to create memory—to change in response to experience and to store those changes in its particular neural networks.

In a young child, the cortex is not yet fully developed; in children younger than three, the neural networks are not mature enough to create what's called linear narrative memory (in other words, a who, what, when, and where memory). However, in lower areas of the brain, other neural networks are processing—and changing as a result of—our earliest experiences. Associations, or memories, are being created in these lower networks, and this has a huge impact on how trauma is stored in the brains of the very young.

If a child experiences abuse, their brain may make an association between the features of the abuser or the circumstances of the abuse—hair color, tone of voice, the music playing in the background—and a sense of fear. The complex and confusing associations can influence behaviors for years; later in life, for example, being served in a restaurant by a brown-haired man who hovers over you while he takes your order may elicit a panic attack. But because there is no firmly embedded cognitive recollection—no linear narrative memory—the panic is often experienced and interpreted as random, independent of any previous experience.

A lifelong set of beliefs and behaviors can emerge when trauma is experienced at a young age. In one of the most serious manifestations, early sexual abuse can poison intimacy, even if the person has no actual recollection of specific instances of abuse.

*Oprah*: Two hundred and seventeen episodes of *The Oprah Winfrey Show* focused on sexual abuse, and I saw a profound through-line for most victims, including myself. When you've been groomed to be compliant, confrontation in any form is uncomfortable because you were never taught that you have the right to say no; in fact, you were taught that you *can't* say no. The sense that you aren't deserving enough to set your own boundaries has been stolen from you. Many people react by burying their feelings of "no" and becoming people pleasers. I fall in that category. For years, I would say yes to things I knew I really did not want to do, or avoid difficult conversations because I could not live with the discomfort of speaking up for myself. I've known other victims of trauma who sabotage situations until someone else says no for them—meaning their relationship ends, a friendship becomes toxic, or they lose a job. This is what I hear you saying when you talk about people who poison intimacy.

But the extreme experiences we've talked about so far—sexual molestation, child abuse, war—aren't the only experiences that can cause trauma. The term can actually apply to a vast spectrum of life events.

For me, there is no better example of this than the story of Kris and Daisy, who first appeared on *The Oprah Winfrey Show* in an episode about children of divorce. At the time, Kris was seven years old. Daisy, his sister, was eleven. Not only had they endured the trauma of their parents' divorce, but it had been several years since they'd had any contact with their mother. Kris was only four when he'd last seen her, and his longing was heartbreaking. He believed that if he could buy a ring for his mother with the money he'd saved, she would come back to him. That broke me wide open.

Daisy's hurt, on the other hand, presented itself as anger. "You're not supposed to have a boyfriend when you're married," she told me, referring to her mother. The woman who was supposed to love her unconditionally and be her greatest teacher had disappeared from her life. Daisy described it as "unbearable."

On the show, rabbi and family therapist M. Gary Neuman told me that for most children, divorce is really like a death. He explained that children don't see their parents as separate people who came together. They see one parent unit within one family unit. So even if divorce is what's best for the family overall, the children feel pieces of themselves being torn away. And if one parent is no longer available, or suddenly introduces a new relationship to the dynamic before the child can develop trust, it impacts the areas of the brain involved in shaping self-worth. The sense of self informs every relationship or decision we make as we move through life. And when children don't feel respected by the decisions of their parents, their beliefs about how they are valued are crushed.

Kris and Daisy were the first children I'd ever heard speak such truth about the trauma of their parents' breaking up. Some people believe that the younger the child, the easier a new relationship is to absorb; Kris and Daisy's story confirmed for me that this isn't true.

I know your research suggests the same. Explain to me from a neurological perspective what happens to a child's brain in that situation.

*Dr. Perry*: When a new relationship enters the picture, two things happen. First, the child—and this is true even of babies—begins asking internally, "Who is this person, and what is this?" Second, they feel the shift of their parent's attention away from them and onto this other person. So you can start to see how destabilizing this is, even without any hostile, aggressive, or abusive stuff going on.

*Oprah*: Meaning even when the relationships are relatively healthy.

*Dr. Perry*: Right. Even if it's a really nice, kind, respectful person entering the child's life, it takes a long time for the child to make sense of the shift and get back to a calm, regulated state. As we'll talk about later, anything new will activate our stress-response systems.

Our default response to novelty is "Uh-oh. What is this?" And until the new thing is proven safe and positive, it will be categorized as a potential threat. For most people, the unknown is one of the major causes of feeling anxious or overwhelmed.

And, of course, it's worse if there is conflict in the relationship. Let's say a young boy is yelled at by his mother's new boyfriend. This experience is processed and stored in the cortex as a narrative—who, what, when, where—memory: "On Monday, the boyfriend came to the house and yelled at me." But it's also stored deeper in the brain. When the boyfriend was yelling, the boy's stress response was activated. The key regulatory systems governed by the lower parts of his brain sped up his heart, increased his muscle tone, and sent signals to his body to prepare for fight or flight. Fear shuts down thinking and amps up feeling, and the boy was afraid. And as his brain is trying to make sense of the whole experience, it's also making a trauma memory.

Later on, when this boy is exposed to a trigger or evocative cue that reminds his brain of that traumatic experience, his heart rate will go up. His body posture will change. The cocktail of hormones in his body will shift. The point is that our body's core regulatory systems can be altered by traumatic experiences. A child exposed to unpredictable or extreme stress will become what we call dysregulated.

*Oprah*: And living in a traumatizing environment causes the child to be continually dysregulated.

*Dr. Perry*: Yes. For instance, if a child sees repeated verbal or emotional or physical abuse of their parent, or experiences abuse directly from a parent's partner, their brain makes connections between all the attributes of the abuser and threat. These associations can influence how the child experiences and interprets relationships as they grow up.

*Oprah*: And that forms what you call a "personal catalog—or the code-book" that shapes the lens through which we perceive the world.

*Dr. Perry*: Absolutely. These early-life associations are incredibly powerful and pervasive. Once, I was working as a consultant to a residential treatment center, where there were about one hundred boys, roughly seven to seventeen years old. All of these children were "state kids"—wards of the state following removal from their family due to abuse or neglect. After struggling in foster care, these boys had been placed in this residential program. They lived in a dorm-like setting, and most of them attended an on-site school.

One boy I worked with was a fourteen-year-old named Samuel. When he was seven, Child Protective Services (CPS) had moved him and his four younger siblings from their home. They had all been neglected, and Samuel had been caring for and protecting the others; when his father drank, Sam was the target of his most violent outbursts. When the children were removed, the younger ones went to a separate foster home. Sam was distraught; he kept running away from foster homes to find them. He'd been in twelve foster homes— and twelve schools—before being placed in the residential setting at age eleven. One of the first things we did was reconnect him with his siblings, setting up weekly calls and monthly visits. Knowing they were safe and loved settled him. Only then could the hard work of healing really start.

For the next three years, Sam made great progress. His social skills improved; he was developing better self-control when frustrated or disappointed; he became more hopeful and focused on the future. Though the chaos in his life had left him three grades behind in school, he was catching up to the point where he was moved up to a new classroom.

Sam's new teacher was energetic, well-liked, experienced—and male. During the first week in the new classroom, Sam had three major outbursts; two of them, directed at the teacher, were so aggressive and violent that Sam had to be physically restrained. This was an extreme intervention for this program and highly unusual behavior for Sam. Unfortunately, it kept happening. The staff was confused and frustrated. Sam was sullen and ashamed.

I sat down with the teacher to review each event, and neither he nor I could see any obvious trigger for the explosive outbursts. I observed Sam's classroom and saw no inappropriate or potentially provocative behavior by the teacher. Yet Sam was clearly agitated anytime the teacher talked with him or tried to give him any help with his work. Proximity was the only possible trigger I saw; the closer the teacher was, the worse Sam's agitation. Over time, the teacher began avoiding any interaction—no eye contact, no verbal encouragement, no smiling. He was disengaging emotionally as well as physically. It was clear these two didn't like each other.

One day when I was talking with Sam about this, his only explanation was, "He hates me. Nothing I do is right." Our session was interrupted by a staff member who reminded Sam that it was almost time for his visit with his father. These visits had to be supervised, and the caseworker had not arrived, so I volunteered to go with Sam.

We went to a conference room, and I sat in the corner waiting for Sam's father to show up. Sam sat at the conference room table stacking checkers. Waiting. His father was late, again. Finally, the door opened, and the father came in and sat down across from Sam. They exchanged awkward greetings and set up to play checkers. For the next ten minutes, maybe ten words were exchanged as they played. Neither looked at the other. The tension was palpable.

My mind drifted as they played. I found myself thinking about my own father. Fishing trips up in Canada, north of Flin Flon. His waking me from a warm slumber at 5 a.m. to get out among the walleye. His putting on his red-checked flannel hunting shirt that had his scent—his special mix of cigar, sweat, and Old Spice. Such a warm and reassuring scent. I was swept with an intense feeling of being safe and loved.

As I surfaced from my daydream, the smell of Old Spice still hung in the room. Could it be? I walked over to the table and bent down between Sam and his father. "How's the game going?"

The father said, "He's winning." I could smell alcohol on his breath and the Old Spice he'd slathered on to hide it. He was supposed to come to see Sam sober.

After the visit ended, I went to see the teacher. He was in his classroom preparing for the next day. "This may seem a bit strange," I said, "but what kind of deodorant do you use?"

"Old Spice. Why?"

I took out a paper and pencil and drew the upside-down triangle model of the brain, and we talked for a minute or two about memory, associations, and triggers. I told him that I thought the scent of Old Spice was an evocative cue for Sam (just like one of Mr. Roseman's evocative cues was explosive sounds). The teacher agreed to change to a scentless deodorant.

Later that afternoon, I asked Sam to sit down with me, and I explained what I thought was making him so uncomfortable and angry with the teacher. I showed Sam the same upside-down triangle brain drawing, and we talked about how our brain makes sense of the world by connecting sights and sounds and smells that "co-occur." He nodded; it made sense to him. He gave me other examples of things he knew pushed his buttons: when someone yelled, he wanted to run and hide; when a bigger person bullied a smaller person, he wanted to attack. I asked if he would be willing to sit down with the teacher and see if we could have a redo on their relationship.

Both Sam and the teacher agreed to give each other another chance. Over the next year, their relationship grew strong, and Sam ended up being a model student in that classroom.

Sam's story illustrates so much about how the brain stores memory. Both Sam and I had experiences earlier in life where our brains made memories connected to the smell of Old Spice. My associations elicited positive feelings; his elicited distress and fear. As we make our way through the world, countless sounds, smells, and images can tap into memories we created earlier in life. These memories may be full-blown recollections of a specific event, or they may be fragments—a feeling, a sense of déjà vu, an impression.

When we meet someone, we form a first impression ("He seems like a really nice guy"), frequently with no apparent information on which to base it. This is because attributes of the person evoke in us something we've previously categorized as familiar and positive. The opposite can happen ("This guy is a complete jerk") if some attribute taps into a previous negative experience.

Our brain catalogs vast amounts of input from our family, community, and culture, along with what is presented to us in the media. As it makes sense of what it's stored, it begins to form a worldview. If we later meet someone with characteristics unlike what we've cataloged, our default response is to be wary, defensive. In turn, if our brains are filled with associations based upon media-driven biases about ideal body type, or racial or cultural stereotypes, for example, we will exhibit implicit biases (and maybe overt bias).

So many phenomena of everyday life are directly linked to this process of the brain making sense of the world by creating associations and making memories. This is why asking "What happened to you?" is so important in understanding what's going on with you now.

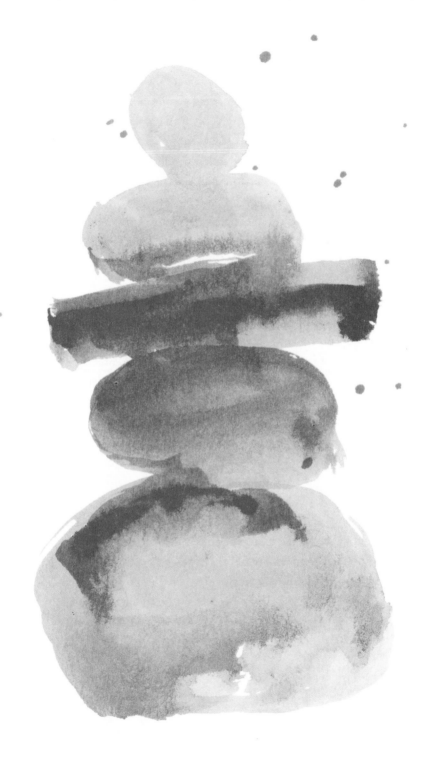

# CHAPTER 2

———

# SEEKING BALANCE

*How much do you think about your heart?*

*Since before you were even born, that miraculous machine has been steadily pumping the energy of life throughout your body. Day in, day out, at least 115,000 beats each day, with the sole purpose of keeping you alive.*

*But beyond the complex physical task of delivering essential nutrients to every cell, tissue, and organ, your heart's pulse also regulates your emotional energy. A strong, even pace can bring a sense of calm. A rapid staccato can panic even the healthiest person.*

*There was a time in my late forties when I noticed a change, a rapid fluttering, in my own heart. I immediately started thinking worst-case scenario. One night I awoke with my heart beating so intensely, I thought for the first time in my life that I was about to die.*

*It took six months before I understood what was happening. A book I found lying on a table outside the studio where we taped* The Oprah Winfrey Show *noted that heart palpitations can be part of menopause. A doctor confirmed that this was true and that my body was indeed undergoing menopausal changes, and I can't tell you how relieved I felt. Relieved and awed. Because for me, those direct messages from my heart were one of the most powerful connections I'd ever made with my unique biosystem. They were proof of what I already believed: that my body is always speaking to me.*

*The same is true for you. From birth, your heart is constantly sending messages about the state of your well-being. It's intimately attuned to the slightest shifts in your physical and emotional health, and when it sends out a warning, every part of you feels the effect.*

*Ever since those episodes with my heart, I've felt deep gratitude for this ever-vigilant internal alarm. In times of stress, its changes in cadence have been a gift.*

*But as I have learned from Dr. Perry, remaining in a constant state of high alert can have devastating effects on your overall physical and emotional health. The correlation between long-term stress and conditions like anxiety, depression, stroke, heart disease, and diabetes is real.*

*I was in my twenties when I was first challenged, in a big way, to regulate my own stress. I'd taken a job as a reporter and was working hundred-hour weeks. I wanted to be a team player, but I could feel myself becoming increasingly out of sync. As I explained earlier, traumatic events in my childhood, including an uprooted family, sexual abuse, and regular beatings, had conditioned me to be a skilled people pleaser, even if it meant completely depleting my own energy. And so, when I felt the stress indicators that my body was sending, I ignored them, choosing instead to soothe myself with the drug that was most easily accessible: food. The more out of rhythm my life became, the more I sought relief to silence the signals.*

*I was tuned in enough to know that I was betraying myself. I knew that I had only a certain amount of energy, and I knew that it needed to be conserved and restored. But it would take decades for me to understand how to live within my own rhythms.*

*Now when I begin to feel overwhelmed, I pull back. I have learned to say no. When I'm around someone who drains me, I put up a barrier—a nonphysical wall that keeps that person's negative energy away.*

*I've also created a sacred personal space, blocking out Sundays as a time of renewal, allowing myself to be with myself, allowing myself simply to be. When this time is interrupted or threatened by someone who invades my state of calm, I become irritable, anxiety-prone, and distressed about making decisions—not the person I want to be in the world. The quickest and most consistent way for me to get back to my own rhythm is to walk in nature. Just focusing on my breath, my steady heartbeat, the stillness of a tree, or the intricacy of a leaf can center me in the wholeness of all things.*

*Music, laughter, dancing (even a party for one), knitting, cooking— finding what naturally soothes you not only regulates your heart and mind, it helps you stay open to the goodness in you and in the world.*

—Oprah

*Oprah*: I remember walking on the OWLAG campus with you, watching the girls dance, sing, and laugh together as they moved from one class to the next. You had been working with the students there for over ten years, and as we looked on, you said something like, "That will help them learn." We ended up talking about why rhythm is so important.

*Dr. Perry*: Rhythm is essential to a healthy body and a healthy mind. Every person in the world can probably think of something rhythmic that makes them feel better: walking, swimming, music, dance, the sound of waves breaking on a beach. . . .

*Oprah*: It's why we rock babies when they cry. We're trying to help them find their own rhythm to help calm them down.

*Dr. Perry*: Exactly, and that will help us calm down, as well. The emotions of people around us are contagious. When our baby is upset, it can make us upset. So we go to the baby and hold her and walk with her. We start with a rhythm that is soothing to us, and if that doesn't work, we slowly shift to a pattern that is regulating for the baby. The baby's response to our efforts shapes the style of the rhythmic soothing we use.

As we grow up, we find our own set of regulating rhythms and activities. For some of us, it is walking. For others, it's doing needlework or riding a bike. Everyone has their go-to options when they feel out of sync, anxious, or frustrated. The common element is rhythm. Rhythm is regulating.

*Oprah*: People use the word *wellness* to mean overall health or balance among mind, body, spirit. But you talk about *regulation*. Help me understand what you mean by that.

*Dr. Perry*: Regulation is also about being in balance. We have many different systems that are continuously monitoring our body and the outside world to make sure we're safe and in balance—that we have enough food, water, oxygen. When we're regulated, these systems have what they need.

Stress is what occurs when a demand or challenge takes us out of balance—away from our regulated "set points." When we get out of balance, we become dysregulated and feel discomfort or distress. When we get back into balance, we feel better. Relief of distress—getting back into balance—activates the reward networks in the brain. We feel pleasure when we get back into balance—from cold to warm, thirsty to quenched, hungry to satiated.

*Oprah*: And regulation is more than a biological concept. In all areas of our lives, we are seeking what we need to be stabilized, balanced, and regulated.

*Dr. Perry*: Yes. Balance is the core of health. We feel and function best when our body's systems are in balance, and when we're in balance with friends, family, community, and nature.

*Oprah*: And what's really important for parents to realize is what you just said—that learning healthy *self-regulation* actually begins in infancy. When babies cry, they're either hungry or thirsty or tired, or their diaper needs changing or they need to be touched. And since they can't feed themselves or change their own diaper, crying is their way to get themselves back into balance—to get their caregiver to do what has to be done in order for them to get back into balance. The problem is when their caregiver doesn't respond. Rather than being put back in balance—regulated—the baby will get more upset.

*Dr. Perry*: Yes. If I get hungry, I get up and make myself a sandwich—I self-regulate. But as you said, the infant has to rely on adults to help her with this. Caregiving adults provide external regulation. Over time, these responsive adults help the child's brain begin to build self-regulating capabilities. And as we've mentioned, one of the most powerful tools we use to help regulate a distressed infant is rhythm.

*Oprah*: Why is that?

*Dr. Perry*: All life is rhythmic. The rhythms of the natural world are embedded in our biological systems. This begins in the womb, when the mother's beating heart creates rhythmic sound, pressure, and vibrations that are sensed by the developing fetus and provide constant rhythmic input to the organizing brain. These experiences create powerful associations—essentially, memories—that connect rhythms of roughly sixty to eighty beats per minute (bpm) to regulation. Sixty to eighty bpm is the average resting heart rate for an adult; it's the rhythm the fetus sensed, and it equates to being in balance, to being warm, full, quenched, safe. After birth, rhythms at these frequencies can comfort and soothe, whereas the loss of rhythm, or high, variable, and unpredictable patterns of sensory input, becomes associated with threat.

When we rock the distressed baby, the rhythmic movement activates this memory of safety. The infant feels more in balance and calms down.

Furthermore, by rocking the baby while also feeding, warming, and loving them, the caring adults strengthen the primary associations between rhythm and regulation. These loving interactions begin to expand the complex "memory" of regulation by mixing in human contact. The caregiver's smell, touch, smile, and voice also become connected with regulation—with safety. The roots of health are rhythm and regulation. When you mix in attentive, responsive, and nurturing caregiving, the roots and trunk of our brain's Tree of Regulation are being organized (see Figure 2).

*Oprah*: So, when you are raised in a nurturing, supportive, caring environment and you cry and someone responds to your needs, you are being regulated. Ultimately, as you grow up with this loving attention, what you describe as the Tree of Regulation grows—and these networks in your brain allow you to regulate yourself and connect to people in healthy relationships.

*Dr. Perry*: Exactly. And this is so important that it's worth a closer look. First, as we've been discussing, we have important neural networks involved in regulation—including our stress-response systems. Second, we have neural networks that are involved in forming and maintaining relationships. Finally, we have neural networks that are involved in "reward"; when these are activated, they give us pleasure. When these three systems begin to wire together, they create our foundational memories; these are the reason that we feel regulated and rewarded when we get signals of acceptance or warmth from another person. A person's capacity to connect, to be regulating and regulated, to reward and be rewarded, is the glue that keeps families and communities together.

*Oprah*: Regulation, relationship, and reward.

*Dr. Perry*: Yes. When the attentive and responsive adult comes to the crying infant, two very important things happen. The baby feels the pleasure of being regulated after being distressed—and also experiences the sight, smell, touch, sound, and movement of human interaction. The loving sensations provided by the adult caregiver start to become associated with pleasure. In thousands of moments, when the caregivers respond to the needs of the infant, the brain is connecting relationship to reward and regulation. And so, when you are an attentive, attuned, and responsive caregiver to these little ones, you're literally weaving together this powerful three-part association—you're building a healthy root system for the Tree of Regulation.

Furthermore, as we talked about earlier, these bonding experiences create the infant's worldview about humans. A consistent, nurturing caregiver builds an internal view that people are safe, predictable, and caring.

*Oprah*: The humans coming to regulate me are not bad. When I need something, it will work out. People are safe and supportive.

*Dr. Perry*: Yes, and that's a remarkable and powerful worldview. We learn that a connection with another person can be rewarding and regulating. It pulls us to engage with our teachers, coaches, classmates. It usually leads to more and more positive human interactions that add to our internal catalog of experience. The brain is a meaning-making machine, always trying to make sense of the world. If our view of the world is that people are good, then we will anticipate good things from people. We project that expectation in our interactions with others and thereby actually elicit good from them. Our internal view of the world becomes a self-fulfilling prophecy; we project what we expect, and that helps elicit what we expect.

Many years ago, I was at Chicago's O'Hare airport in the winter on my way to an academic conference. It was snowing, and all the flights were delayed. The gate area was filled with frustrated people, including an older gentleman sitting next to me. He was wearing a very expensive suit and a Rolex watch, and his frustration was clear. Each time the gate agent announced a further delay, he would mutter with fury and angrily snap his newspaper before reading some more.

*Figure 2*

## TREE OF REGULATION

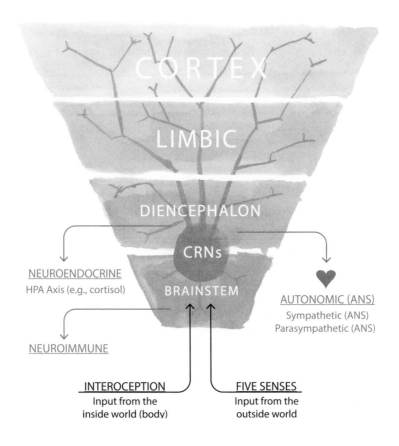

---

**Note: HPA = Hypothalamic-Pituitary-Adrenal Axis;**
**ANS = Autonomic Nervous System; CRNs = Core Regulatory Networks**

---

The Tree of Regulation is comprised of a set of neural networks our body uses to help us process and respond to stress. We tend to use the word *stress* in negative ways, but stress is merely a demand on one or more of our body's many physiological systems. Hunger, thirst, cold, working out, a promotion at work: All are stressors, and stress is an essential and positive part of normal development; it's a key element in learning, mastering new skills, and building resilience. The key factor in determining whether stress is positive or destructive is the pattern of stress, as shown in Figure 3.

We have a set of core regulatory networks (CRNs), or neural systems, originating in the lower parts of the brain and spreading throughout the whole brain, that work together to keep us regulated in the face of various stressors.

Collectively, the branches of this Tree of Regulation direct or influence all functions of the brain (like thinking and feeling) and the body (impacting your heart, stomach, lungs, pancreas, and more). They are trying to keep everything in equilibrium, everything regulated, everything in balance.

I was watching a tired-looking young couple take turns following their daughter, a toddler, as she explored around the gate. For hours, as the stranded passengers grew more and more irritated, the toddler kept smiling, exploring and touching everything she saw.

At one point, when the gate agent came out and announced another delay, the man next to me burst from his seat, almost ran to the agent, and loudly demanded to see her supervisor. "I'm a gold medallion traveler, and I know people on the Board. I'm due in Cleveland for a very important meeting. . . ." The whole gate fell silent as his rant continued.

The poor gate agent simply looked out the window, pointed to the heavy snow falling, and said, "I'm sorry, sir. We are doing our best, but we can't control the weather." The man huffed back to his seat.

Now, in my working model of the world, rude, entitled men treating people poorly are jerks, but when I glanced over at the little girl, her head was cocked as if she were trying to figure out why everyone had gotten quiet when this man talked. Her working model of the world was that people are good. So whatever else this man might be, he was good, too.

She walked right over and stood before him; she put her sticky little hands on his knees and smiled. He frowned and snapped his paper up to read, right in front of her face. My worldview was reinforced: He's even mean to little children? Super jerk.

The little girl paused. Then, clearly thinking that this was a game—because people are good, right?—she smiled and ripped the paper down, beaming at who she thought would be her new playmate.

*Oh, man,* I thought. *This is bad.* But I was wrong. And she was right.

She smiled her big smile. And, shaking his head in defeat, he smiled back. Her "goodness projected" was contagious. She drew the best from this man, and her worldview was reinforced. For the next thirty minutes, the two of them played together as her parents looked on; he even got down on his hands and knees—expensive suit be damned—to give her a horsey ride around the dirty, crowded gate.

She elicited what she projected, thanks to an internalized view of the world that came from thousands of loving moments when her parents, family, and caregivers were present, attentive, and responsive in loving ways.

*Oprah*: But what happens when a baby doesn't get those positive, nurturing responses? Say, if a mom is on her own with no help, or depressed, or in a violent relationship? She may really want to be a loving, responsive parent, but is that possible under those circumstances?

*Dr. Perry*: This is one of the central problems in our society; we have too many parents caring for children with inadequate supports. The result is what you would expect. An overwhelmed, exhausted, dysregulated parent will have a hard time regulating a child consistently and predictably. This can impact the child in two really important ways.

First, it affects the development of the child's stress-response systems (see Figure 3). If the hungry, cold, scared infant is inconsistently responded to—and regulated—by the overwhelmed caregiver, this creates an inconsistent, prolonged, and unpredictable activation of the child's stress-response systems. The result is a sensitization of these important systems.

In prolonged cases of trauma, the CRNs of the Tree of Regulation change and adapt so that they can better cope with the current challenge. The system works hard to keep you in balance, but it can be difficult and exhausting. And in these long-term cases, even when the challenge passes, the change in these systems persists. The hypervigilance of a boy living with domestic violence scanning his home for any sign of threat is very adaptive; in a classroom, this can prevent the child from paying attention to the teacher and result in the child being labeled with attention deficit disorder (ADHD), which is maladaptive.

The second major problem has to do with that process of creating connections about relationships. If, while the infant is creating her working model of the world, the caregiver responds in unpredictable ways, or is episodically rough, frustrated, cold, or absent, the child begins to create a different sort of worldview.

We had a project working with a preschool where we were observing student-teacher interactions. In one of the classrooms, there was a young, enthusiastic, and very nurturing teacher. At the beginning of the year, this teacher warmly greeted each child, gave them a hug and a big smile. All during the day, this teacher interacted with the children in very attentive ways.

We noticed that one little girl avoided this teacher's physical affection and never made eye contact. When the teacher hugged her, she simply stood still and didn't reciprocate. Eventually we learned that this child had a very overwhelmed, depressed mother and that no other adults were in the household.

As time went by, the teacher continued to be warm and effusive with the other children, but week by week, the positive overtures to this withdrawn, sad girl decreased. You can imagine that this girl's worldview was *I'm not that important; you can't really trust people.*

About a month into the school year, the class was doing an activity when the little girl raised her hand for help; it was the first time she'd ever reached out that way. She held her hand high. Waved it. But the teacher was fully engaged with a group of children at another table and didn't notice. The teacher was laughing and smiling with the other children. The little girl watched for a few moments, then slowly lowered her hand. For the rest of the year, she never asked for help again.

After the project was over, we showed the video clip to the teacher, who started to cry. She felt terrible guilt. There was no

*Figure 3*

## PATTERNS OF STRESS ACTIVATION

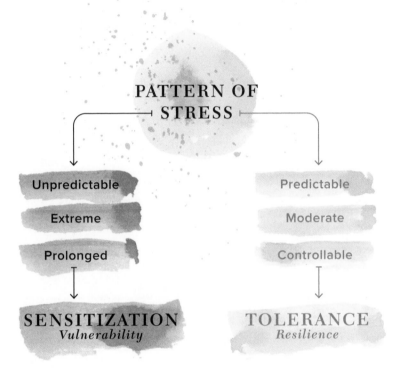

The long-term effects of stress are determined by the pattern of stress activation. When the stress-response systems are activated in unpredictable or extreme or prolonged ways, the systems becomes overactive and overly reactive—in other words, sensitized. Over time, this can lead to functional vulnerability, and since the stress-response systems collectively reach all parts of the brain and body, a cascade of risk in emotional, social, mental, and physical health occurs. In contrast, predictable, moderate, and controllable activation of the stress-response systems, such as that seen with developmentally appropriate challenges in education, sport, music, and so forth, can lead to a stronger, more flexible stress-response capability—i.e., resilience.

intention to ignore this girl, but we all require some reciprocal social feedback to stay engaged. The little girl's working model of the world—*I don't matter*—projected into the classroom and became a self-fulfilling prophecy. We elicit from the world what we project into the world; but what you project is based upon what *happened to you* as a child.

*Oprah*: So, because this little girl may not have had her basic needs met earlier in her life, because her mother was overwhelmed, alone, exhausted, and depressed, and therefore unable to be "present, attentive, attuned, and responsive," as you say, the child is out of balance. And if this pattern of care develops into outright neglect— where the fundamental needs are ignored for longer and longer periods of time, or those cries for help go unmet or are responded to with anger or punishment—the child is living with constant distress. In either situation, she is out of balance.

*Dr. Perry*: Absolutely. And probably the most important aspect of this is the pattern of stress activation. If the parent is consistent, predictable, and nurturing, the stress-response systems become resilient. If the stress-response systems are activated in prolonged ways or chaotic ways, as in cases of abuse or neglect, they become sensitized and dysfunctional.

Though we're generally not aware of it, we are continually sensing and processing information from the outside world; based upon this input, our brain and body respond in ways that help keep us connected, alive, and thriving. When we are pushed out of equilibrium—out of balance—we have a set of stress-response systems that will be activated to help us.

Most people are familiar with the term "fight or flight." This refers to a set of responses that can kick in when we are afraid. Your brain will focus your attention on the potential threat, shutting down unnecessary mental processes (like reflecting on the meaning of life or daydreaming about an upcoming vacation). Your sense of time collapses to the moment. Your heart rate goes up, sending blood to your muscles in preparation, potentially, for fleeing or fighting. Adrenaline pumps through your body. This response is activating your body.

As we'll talk more about later, this "arousal" response is not the only way we can respond to a threat. Imagine a situation where you are too small to win a fight and unable to run away. In this case, the brain and the rest of the body prepare for injury. Your heart rate goes down. You release your body's own painkiller—opioids. You disengage from the external world and psychologically flee into your inner world. Time seems to slow. You may feel like you are in a movie, or floating and watching things happen to you. This is all part of another adaptive capability, called dissociation. For babies and very young children, dissociation is a very common adaptive strategy; fighting or fleeing won't protect you, but "disappearing" might. You learn to escape into your inner world. You dissociate. And over time, your capacity to retreat to that inner world—safe, free, in control—increases. A key part of that sensitized ability to dissociate is to be a people pleaser. You comply with what others want. You find yourself doing things to avoid conflict, to ensure that the other person in the interaction is pleased, as well as gravitating toward various regulating, but dissociative, activities.

Finding balance can be an exhausting challenge for anyone with trauma-altered stress-response systems. The search to avoid the pain of distress can lead to extreme, ultimately destructive, methods of regulation.

*Oprah*: One of the most raw conversations I've had about the struggle to find relief from emotional imbalance was with the British actor and comedian Russell Brand. At the time, he'd been sober for eleven years, but he'd recently published a powerful essay about how he continued to think about heroin nearly every day. "Drugs and alcohol are not my problem," he wrote. "Reality is my problem, drugs and alcohol are my solution."

Russell told me that as a child, he felt alienated from the people around him. He was raised by a single mother with very little money, and he described himself as confused, lonely, and at a loss as to how to handle his feelings. There were points in his life when he could "not distinguish between where he ended and the pain began," and he developed dangerous habits including compulsive eating, an "infatuation" with pornography, and eventually a devastating addiction to drugs.

"I couldn't cope with being me," Russell said. Yet even during some of his darkest moments, he said he often felt gratitude for the respite drugs provided from what he called an overwhelming "internal storm."

On the sixteenth anniversary of his sobriety, Russell went on social media to credit his in-patient recovery treatment, support groups, and mentors. He said, "I have freedom now, and you can have freedom too."

The spiritual teacher Gary Zukav has said, "When you find an addiction, do not be ashamed. Be joyful. You have found something that you have come to this Earth to heal. When you confront and heal an addiction, you are doing the deepest spiritual work that you can do on this Earth."

All this is by way of saying that we've known for years that there is a correlation between drug addiction and trauma, but the death toll just keeps rising. Dr. Perry, through your work with trauma victims, you've found that most people are not taking drugs for the reasons that we think. It's not about self-indulgence and pleasure-seeking, or even a method to escape life in general, as much as it is about avoiding the pain and distress of dysregulation. True?

*Dr. Perry*: So often when we ask, "What happened?" we find a history of developmental trauma. Most people with "developmental adversity" are chronically dysregulated—they tend to be wound up, anxious. Sometimes they feel like they are jumping out of their skin—or, as Russell Brand described it so well, the internal storm. As we will talk more about in a bit, their CRNs are sensitized.

If you grow up in a household or community characterized by unpredictability, chaos, and ongoing threat, you will very likely end up with altered stress-response systems. This is especially true if the abuse, chaos, or exposure to violence took place in the home, and the very adults who were supposed to be nurturing and protecting you were the source of the pain, chaos, fear, or abuse.

Remember what we said about the pattern of stress activation: Even in the absence of major traumatic events, unpredictable stress and the lack of control that goes with it are enough to make our stress-response systems sensitized—overactive and overly reactive—creating the internal storm.

And also remember that humans are emotionally "contagious"; we sense the distress of others. Imagine a child in a home with a frustrated, angry father who has no job prospects, is disrespected in the community due to his status or skin color, and comes home feeling impotent, defeated. This parent's internal storm becomes the home's storm. His chaos becomes the home's chaos. He may use alcohol or a drug to manage his distress. But a drug-using parent, a drunk, overwhelmed, frustrated parent is going to create a climate of fear for their children. As much as they may want to protect the children from their distress, and as much as they love their children, the mess is made. The children grow up internalizing this; they are incubated in terror.

And as these children get older and are introduced to drugs or alcohol themselves, they may discover that they can feel a quiet they have never experienced; the pleasure that comes from the relief of

*Figure 4*

# FILLING OUR REWARD BUCKET

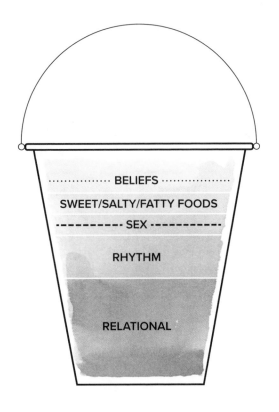

A

Activation of key neural networks in the brain can produce the sense of pleasure or reward. These reward circuits can be activated in multiple ways, including relief of distress (e.g., using Alcohol to self-medicate or Rhythm to regulate the anxiety produced by a stress-response system that's been altered by trauma); positive human interactions (Relational); direct activation of the reward systems using various drugs of abuse such as cocaine or heroin (Drugs); eating Sweet-Salty-Fatty Foods (SSF foods); and behaviors consistent with your values or beliefs (Beliefs).

Each day we need to fill our "reward bucket." The darker dashed line is a minimal level of reward that we need to feel adequately regulated and rewarded; if our daily set of rewards falls below this, we feel distressed. If we get above the upper,

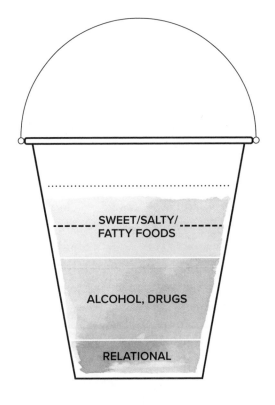

**B**

black-dotted line, we feel fulfilled and regulated. Each of us does this in a somewhat individualized way.

Many of us have opportunities for healthy rewards: lots of positive human interactions through work, worship, or volunteering that are consistent with our values and beliefs, for example (A). But a lack of strong relationships and connection can make an individual more vulnerable to overuse of other, less healthy forms of reward (B). A healthy combination of rewards (e.g., lots of positive human interactions, doing work consistent with your values, integrating healthy rhythm and sexuality into your day, staying regulated in healthy ways) can help decrease the pull toward any single, unhealthy form of reward such as substance use or overeating.

distress becomes a powerful reward. Remember: Relief of distress gives pleasure. They are relaxed for the first time in their lives. The pull to go back and use again is very powerful, though it's affected by how dysregulated you are, and by the nature and strength of the other sources of reward in your life. Every day we "fill our reward bucket" with various sources of reward—and not every day is the same (see Figure 4). Some days will be rich with friends and family; other days you may fill your "reward bucket" by volunteering at a local food kitchen. And some days, we are left empty, unfulfilled. Many of us found it harder to "fill up" during the COVID-19 pandemic; people reported more anxiety and depression, and many people used some of the less healthy forms of reward to fill that void.

The challenge with activating our reward circuits is that the pleasure fades. The feeling of reward is short-lived. Think how long the pleasure of eating a potato chip lasts. A few seconds. Then you want another. Same with a hit of nicotine from a cigarette. Or even the smile of a loved one. It feels so good in the moment, and we can recall it and get a little pleasure, but the intense sense of reward fades. So each day we are pulled to refill our reward bucket.

The healthiest way to do this is through relationships. Connectedness regulates and rewards us. Yet when substance abuse is involved, it can push loved ones away. And many interventions used to deal with substance abuse are punitive and increase distress. The pull to use gets stronger. Disconnection, marginalization, demonizing, and punishing only make the problems of substance abuse worse. The cycle of dysregulation, self-medication, relational disruption, lack of reward leads to more substance abuse. And the spiral continues.

But here's what's interesting about drug use: For people who are pretty well-regulated, whose basic needs have been met, who have other healthy forms of reward, taking a drug will have some impact, but the pull to come back and use again and again is not as powerful.

It may be a pleasurable feeling, but you're not necessarily going to become addicted.

Addiction is complex. But I believe that many people who struggle with drug and alcohol abuse are actually trying to self-medicate due to their developmental histories of adversity and trauma.

*Oprah*: It's interesting to hear you say that, because I know lots of people who take drugs for their anxiety, whereas I have found medications like that just put me to sleep. Because my internal baseline is already so calm, when I take something that's supposed to just relax me, I doze off.

*Dr. Perry*: Right. You probably have friends who take the same amount that puts you to sleep.

*Oprah*: In some cases, they're taking twice as much. And I'm thinking, *How is everybody not just asleep?* But if your baseline stress response is already elevated, you need more anxiety medication to get below your base. So even though people may not appear to be in a state of high alert or anxiety, they are biologically revved up.

*Dr. Perry*: Yes, and the drug soothes that. But when it comes to finding solutions to substance abuse and freedom from it, we will never truly solve the problem until we begin to focus on what happened to them.

*Oprah*: Yes. *What happened to you?* Always the question to ask first.

*Dr. Perry*: This is why a developmentally informed, trauma-aware perspective is so important for all of our systems impacted by or dealing with substance use and dependence—education, mental health, health, law enforcement, juvenile and criminal justice, family courts.

It is impossible to find any part of our society where this is not an issue. We have such good intentions, and we have good people, and we're spending a lot of money, but we're ineffective because we are not understanding the underlying mechanisms that make someone vulnerable to chronic substance use.

*Oprah*: We need to understand that victims of trauma are more prone to all forms of addiction because their baseline of stress is different.

*Dr. Perry*: It comes back to dysregulation. There's always a pull to regulate, to seek comfort, to fill that reward bucket. But it turns out that the most powerful form of reward is relational. Positive interactions with people are rewarding and regulating. Without connection to people who care for you, spend time with you, and support you, it is almost impossible to step away from any form of unhealthy reward and regulation. This includes alcohol overuse, drug overuse, eating too much sweet and salty food, porn, cutting, or spending hours and hours on video games. Connectedness counters the pull of addictive behaviors. It is the key.

CHAPTER 3

———

# HOW WE WERE LOVED

I sat in the darkened room watching the mother, Gloria, and her three-year-old daughter, Tilly, through a one-way mirror. They were doing great together. Gloria was tracking with Tilly's cues, much more in sync than in previous visits. Both appeared more comfortable with each other. Over the two years I had been watching their visits together, there had been so much positive change.

On my left was Tilly's new Child Protective Services (CPS) case-worker, her fifth over the last two years. On my right was Mama P, the child's foster mother. I'd known Mama P for years. She was a loving woman with an endless reserve of positive energy. She had fostered dozens of children; each was special to her, each loved. Mama P probably taught me more about trauma and healing than anyone.

Gloria had been removed from her family when she was six. She struggled as she grew up in the child protective system, bouncing from foster home to foster home, school to school, community to community. Gloria had multiple complex social, emotional, and physical health problems related to her many traumatic experiences. Unfortunately, she'd been misunderstood by everyone: her therapists, foster caretakers, caseworkers, judges, teachers. Twenty years ago, awareness of the impact of trauma wasn't very high.

By age eighteen, when Gloria "aged out of the system," she was using a variety of drugs to self-medicate her pain. On her nineteenth birthday, she was eight months pregnant and homeless. By her twentieth, she had an infant daughter, no support, no family, no work. Ultimately, the child protective system removed Tilly. Fortunately, Tilly was sent straight to Mama P.

Over the next two years, Mama P helped both Gloria and Tilly. She was attentive and nurturing, creating a safe and stable home for Tilly. And she invited Gloria to be present and involved in Tilly's life as long as she wasn't using or drinking. Mama P realized that Gloria needed as much safe and stable nurturing as Tilly; she realized that Gloria was a young, unloved child in a woman's body. In the beginning,

Gloria didn't engage much. But after nine months or so, she accepted our offer to get clinical help for her trauma-related problems.

By now, both Tilly and Gloria had grown up significantly. It was getting close to the time when Gloria would be able to care for Tilly on her own. But for that to happen, CPS had to make that recommendation to the court. This observed visit was part of the CPS "reunification" plan.

We three sat silently, watching Tilly and Gloria. After about ten minutes of play, Gloria reached into her coat pocket and pulled out some candy. I could feel the CPS caseworker stiffen. "She is not supposed to bring candy to these sessions." On my other side, I could feel Mama P make herself bigger in response to the caseworker's words. I quietly put my hand on Mama P's, trying to reassure her. She was very protective of both Gloria and Tilly.

Tilly was prediabetic. In the first year of treatment, we'd noticed that Gloria, with so few relationship tools, used candy to make Tilly "happy." We came to understand that this was the primary way in which Gloria's foster caregivers had managed her when she was young; getting candy was the closest Gloria got to being loved. Our brains develop as a reflection of the world we grow up with. You love others the way you've been loved. Gloria was merely showing love to her daughter the best way she knew.

The caseworker continued, "She knows that she is not supposed to do that. This child is prediabetic. This is abusive."

"No," I said. "It's sugar-free candy." Clearly, this caseworker, new to Tilly and likely dealing with sixty other cases, had not read the most recent reports.

"How do you know that?"

"I gave them to her before the session." I could feel Mama smiling.

A year earlier, in a team meeting where we were trying to figure out the best way to balance Tilly's prediabetic condition with Gloria's impulse to use candy to show love, one of my clinical team members wanted to admonish Gloria. He suggested searching her before visits and prohibiting contact if she snuck candy to Tilly. Mama P disagreed. "That poor mother is doing the best she can. Let her give her daughter some candy. That is all she knows. You will not make her a better parent by punishing or shaming her. If we want her to be a more loving parent, we need to be more loving to her."

So instead of admonishing Gloria, we simply had her switch to sugar-free candy, and taught her about nutrition and diabetes. And, of course, Mama P made sure that Gloria and Tilly both got lots of love.

We explained this to the new caseworker, and together we created a transitional plan for reunification with lots of support for both Gloria and Tilly. Gloria got her GED and went to community college to study nursing. Mama P stayed active in their little family. Rather than undermine a mother doing the best she could, we kept showing Gloria and Tilly love, and how to love.

One of the most remarkable properties of our brain is its capacity to change and adapt to our individual world. Neurons and neural networks actually make physical changes when stimulated; this is called neuroplasticity. The way they become stimulated is through our particular experiences: The brain changes in a "use dependent" way. The neural networks involved in piano playing, for example, will make changes when activated by a child practicing her piano. These experience-dependent changes translate into better piano playing. This aspect of neuroplasticity—repetition leads to change—is well known and is why practice in sports, arts, and academics can lead to improvement.

A key principle of neuroplasticity is specificity. In order to change any part of the brain, that specific part of the brain must be activated. If you want to learn to play the piano, you can't simply read about piano playing, or watch and listen to YouTube clips of other people playing piano. You must put your hands on the keys and play; you have to stimulate the parts of the brain involved in piano playing in order to change them.

*This principle of "specificity" applies to all brain-mediated func-tions, including the capacity to love. If you have never been loved, the neural networks that allow humans to love will be undeveloped, as in Gloria's case. The good news is that with use, with practice, these capabilities can emerge. Given love, the unloved can become loving.*

—Dr. Perry

*Oprah*: If I were to count the number of people I've interviewed—and believe me, I've tried—it would be over fifty thousand. And in nearly forty years of conversations, beginning with my early years working in Nashville, through *The Oprah Winfrey Show* and up to today, one common denominator has never changed: All of us want to know that what we do, what we say, and who we are matters.

Like clockwork, whether it's the President of the United States, Beyoncé in all her Beyoncé-ness, a mother sharing a painful secret, or a convicted criminal in search of forgiveness, at the end of any interview, the person sitting across from me asks, "How did I do?" as they scan my face for a reaction. "Was I okay?" they always ask. The longing to be accepted and affirmed in their truth is the same for everyone. And beyond science, I know it boils down to this: how you were loved.

*Dr. Perry*: Yes, belonging and being loved are core to the human experience. We are a social species; we are meant to be in community—emotionally, socially, and physically interconnected with others. If you look at the fundamental organization and functioning of the human body, including the brain, you will see that so much of it is intended to help us create, maintain, and manage social interactions. We are relational creatures.

And the capacity to be connected in meaningful and healthy ways is shaped by our earliest relationships. Love, and loving caregiving, is the foundation of our development. *What happened to you* as an infant has a profound impact on this capacity to love and be loved.

*Oprah*: The word *love* gets thrown around a lot. But really, the key is how you were given care; how your specific needs were met. I'm thinking of what we talked about earlier with regulation. The baby will be hungry or cold—out of balance. And when the baby cries, expressing need, the caregiver comes and "regulates" the child.

*Dr. Perry*: The caregiver coming to meet the needs of the infant is key. To the newborn, *love is action;* it is the attentive, responsive, nurturing care that adults provide. A parent may truly love his child, but if he is sitting at a computer posting on social media about how much he loves his child while the infant is in another room, awake, hungry, and crying, the infant experiences no love. To the infant, skin-to-skin warmth, the smell of the parent, the sights and sounds of her caregivers, the attentive and responsive caregiver's actions—that becomes *love.*

The thousands of these loving, responsive interactions shape the developing brain of the infant. These loving moments literally build the foundation of the organizing brain.

The pattern of stress activation created when the infant gets hungry, thirsty, or cold, and the caregiver meets their need and gets them back in balance, is the *resilience-building* pattern we talked about earlier (see Chapter 2, Figure 3). The moderately stressed infant cries, the cries bring the responsive nurturing adult to regulate them, and because the adults are present, attentive, and responsive, their loving behaviors become predictable. *When I feel hungry, I cry and they come and feed me.* The infant begins to associate these responsive people with pleasure, sustenance, warmth; her view of the world is being shaped. Remember our little girl in the airport? *People are good.* It is through these interactions that the child's worldview is built, and depending upon the quality and pattern of the caregiver's responses, will build resilience or contribute to a sensitized, vulnerable child.

*Oprah*: In every single interaction, there is a moment when we all wonder, *Do you see me? Do you hear me?* Children know from birth whether their caregiver's eyes light up when they enter a room. They sense and respond to tenderness, playfulness, compassion, and patience. They know the true feeling of quality time. They know they are loved.

*Dr. Perry*: And in turn, these caregiving interactions help build the infant's capacity to love. The attentive, loving behaviors grow the neural networks that allow us to feel love, and then act in loving ways toward others. If you are loved, you learn to love. Caring for the infant in this loving way also changes the brain of the caregiving adult. These interactions regulate and reward both child and caregiver.

The capacity to love is at the core of the success of humankind. The reason we've survived on this planet is that we've been able to form and maintain effective groups. Isolated and disconnected, we are vulnerable. In community, we can protect one another, cooperatively hunt and gather, share with the dependents of our family, our clan. Relational glue keeps our species alive, and love is relational superglue.

*Oprah*: The way you treat a child, from the time that child is born, is what sets them up to either succeed or struggle. What you are really saying is, how you were loved informs the way your important neural networks are shaped, especially those core regulatory networks we talked about earlier.

*Dr. Perry*: Yes, that's right. There is a lot of complexity to that, but attentive, loving interactions organize and shape the CRNs. This creates a foundation for health that will be built upon as the child grows up.

Think of it like building a house. The foundation is put in place first, then the framing, then the flooring and wiring and plumbing— all of it before the house can be occupied. As we've said before, the brain also develops from the bottom up. The lowest networks, those that make up the CRNs, develop first, starting in the womb, and the functions they mediate and modulate show up first during our development. The healthy newborn, for example, can regulate body temperature and basic respiration but isn't capable of abstract reasoning. Even sleep isn't really well organized yet; motor movement is uncoordinated. Over time, however, the baby can stand, the toddler will talk, the child will begin to plan, and so forth. The functions related to the middle and then top parts of the brain begin to fully organize (see Figure 1).

The developmental process is very front-loaded, meaning that the majority of brain growth and organization takes place in the first years of life. Now, this doesn't mean that the brain won't change after early childhood, but early life experiences do have a very powerful impact on how we develop.

Let's look at the Tree of Regulation again (see Figure 2). Collectively, the core regulatory networks can reach every part of the developing brain. In fact, the signals the brain receives from the CRNs play a major role in how each of its areas develops. If the CRNs are normally organized and regulated, their signals will result in healthy development of the important higher areas (e.g., limbic and cortex). But if anything disrupts or alters the CRNs, all of the brain and body systems they influence can be adversely affected.

There are three types of "developmental adversity" that will predictably alter the CRNs and cause widespread problems. The first is disruption that happens before birth, such as prenatal exposure to drugs, alcohol, or extreme maternal distress (of the kind that can occur with domestic violence, for example). The second is some form of disruption of the early interactions between infant and caregiver; if these are chaotic, inconsistent, rough, aggressive, or absent, the stress-response systems will develop in abnormal ways. The third is any sensitizing pattern of stress. This can result from a host of circumstances, many of which we will talk about later in more detail; the basic idea is that anything that can cause unpredictable, uncontrollable, or extreme and prolonged activations of the stress response will result in an overactive and overly reactive stress response (see Figure 5).

## Figure 5

## STATE-REACTIVITY CURVE

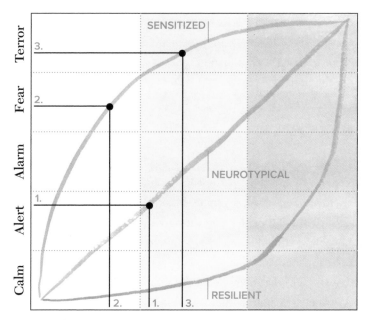

Daily challenge    Moderate stress    Distress – threat

When a challenge or stressor occurs, it will push us out of balance, and an internal stress response will be activated to get us back in balance. With no significant stressors—no internal needs (hunger, thirst, etc.) unmet and no external complexity or threat—we will be in a state of calm. As challenges and stress increase, our internal state will shift, from alert to terror (see Figure 6).

In someone with *neurotypical* stress-response systems, there is a linear relationship between the degree of stress and the shift in internal state (straight diagonal line). For example, in the face of a moderate stressor (1), a proportional activation will put the individual in an active alert state. If an individual has a *sensitized* stress response (top curve) caused by their history of trauma, even the most basic daily challenges (2) will induce a state of fear. Someone with a sensitized stress response (3) will respond to even moderate stress with a terror response. This overreactivity contributes to their emotional, behavioral, and physical health problems.

*Oprah*: So how you were loved is much more complex than simply saying, "You weren't handled with affection as a child; therefore, you will be sad." What you're really saying is that if you were treated aggressively, or if there was chaotic or neglectful caregiving, or if you weren't held as a child, your brain could be biologically affected.

*Dr. Perry*: Exactly. Childhood experiences literally impact the biology of the brain.

*Oprah*: And as a result, it will affect how you function for the rest of your life.

*Dr. Perry*: It can. Our earliest developmental experiences, particularly touch and other relational-based sensory cues, including the caregiver's smell and the way they rock the infant, the songs they hum when feeding the infant, any unique movement in the way they respond to the infant when it's needy—all of these things are organizing experiences that help create the infant's "worldview," the "codebook" we talked about earlier.

Again, think of building a house. The fetal brain is developing so rapidly, it's like putting in the foundation of a building. In the first couple of months after you're born, it's like putting up the framing. In the first year, all of your interactions with others are adding the wiring and plumbing. All of these are really important parts of building the house. It's not fully organized yet, but most of the major characteristics of the building are put in place. A two-year-old child is not yet fully developed, but the foundational structures and systems are there, and these will be the basis for future development.

With a house, if you do a bad job with the foundation, put in shoddy wiring and plumbing but decorate it with beautiful flooring and furniture, the core defects in the house may not be visible as you first walk through. But these early construction issues will lead to problems later on. The same is true with a young child. Really, every aspect of human functioning is influenced by early developmental experiences—both when there are consistent, predictable, and loving interactions and when there is chaos, threat, unpredictability, or lack of love.

*Oprah*: Yes! How were you loved—it makes all the difference. In all the conversations I've had, my experience has been that dysfunction shows up in direct proportion to how you were or were not loved. Did you get what you needed to thrive?

*Dr. Perry*: Love, given and felt, is dependent upon the ability to be present, attentive, attuned, and responsive to another human being. This glue of humanity has been essential to the survival of our species—and to the health and happiness of the individual. And this ability is based upon *what happened to you,* primarily as a young child.

*Oprah*: As we're talking about this, I'm thinking back to when I was asked to list my favorite moments from *The Oprah Winfrey Show*. It wasn't so much the big shows, the surprises or the famous guests—it was the quiet conversations. And the Cheerios girl is always one of the first to come to mind.

An eleven-year-old named Kate and her older brother, Zach, joined me on the show a few months after they'd lost their mother, Kathleen. They told me that prior to her death, their parents decided to spend Kathleen's last months taking trips together as a family. I asked Kate what her favorite moment from that time had been. Her answer was, for me, a huge *Aha.*

"One day when I came back from swimming," Kate told me, "my mom was in bed. She said, 'Kate, would you get me a bowl of cereal?' I said, 'Sure.' Then, one week before she died, I was in my parents' room. I said, 'Mom, would you wake me up if you go downstairs to get a bowl of cereal?' She said she would. So at 2:00 in the morning, we had a bowl of Cheerios together." The family had been everywhere together, but what stayed with Kate was an everyday intimate moment between a mother and a daughter.

*Dr. Perry*: That's a wonderful example of the glue of love. It is in the small moments, when we feel the other person fully present, fully engaged, connected, and accepting, that we make the most powerful, enduring bonds.

*Oprah*: We went back and checked on Kate twenty years after that cereal moment. She let us know that while she has faced painful personal struggles, she still believes strongly in the profound power of connection during life's little yet transcendent moments—these safe, nurturing, and fully present moments you're talking about.

*Dr. Perry*: I love this story because it makes a really important point about these special moments—that the most powerful and enduring human interactions are often very brief. You can spend hours with someone, but if you are not present and attentive, the hours are less powerful than these brief cereal moments.

*Oprah*: And when you don't get your cereal moments—if you are a child born in an environment of chaos, confusion, violence, or disruption, with no normalcy or regularity—you are being set up to fail. Because the networks in your brain don't organize in the way they should.

*Dr. Perry*: Correct. That can result in a weaker foundation or miswiring that creates risk for the rest of life. A big part of the vulnerability will come from the way chaotic and unpredictable caregiving influences the developing stress-response systems to become sensitized.

*Oprah*: Explain how that happens. What does that look like?

*Dr. Perry*: Well, let's talk some more about neuroplasticity—remember, neuroplasticity is basically the changeability of the brain. One of the key principles of neuroplasticity is that the *pattern of activation* makes a big difference in how a neural network changes.

For example, moderate, predictable, and controllable activation of our stress-response systems leads to a more flexible, stronger stress-response capability (see Figure 3) that lets a person demonstrate resilience in the face of more extreme stressors. It's kind of like weight lifting for our stress-response systems; we exercise the system to make it stronger. The more we face moderate challenges and succeed, the more capable we are of facing bigger challenges. This is something we see in sports, performing arts, clinical practice, firefighting, teaching—almost any human endeavor; experience can improve performance. This is why stress is not something to be afraid of or avoided. It is the controllability, pattern, and intensity of stress that can cause problems.

Unfortunately, for far too many people, the pattern of stress activation is unpredictable, uncontrollable, prolonged, or extreme.

Many years ago, I was called to see a child in the hospital, a thirteen-year-old boy named Jesse. He was in a coma following a head injury that resulted from a fight with his foster father.

Jesse was born to a family that had a multigenerational history of sexual abuse, sexual exploitation, involvement in trafficking, and prostituting children. When Jesse was five, a police investigation found that his parents had been prostituting him.

Jesse was removed from his home and placed in foster care. He bounced around the system and, after three failed placements, ended up in a foster home that specialized in high-needs children. The foster parents also cared for nine other children. Many of them had profound developmental problems—delayed language development, explosive and aggressive behaviors, fecal smearing. All had been sent to this home due to "uncontrollable" behaviors; this family was regarded as having a good track record with "difficult" children.

As it turns out, this family "managed" the children with terror and abuse. Food was withheld for minor "infractions," physically abusive punishment was routine, forced exercise was used to exhaust the children, "misbehaving" children were forced to sleep outside in a chicken coop. The refrigerator was locked so the children couldn't "steal" food; the family's biological teenage children were encouraged to participate in the humiliation and physical abuse of the foster children.

Jesse tried to run away from this hell several times. They took away his shoes and clothes at night to try to stop him. He ran anyway but was always caught and brought back. Once, in winter, running barefoot down a country road in nothing but his underwear, he was picked up by a county deputy sheriff. Jesse told the deputy about the abuse. The deputy told Jesse to stop lying about the good people who had the generosity to bring him into their home. That night he was forced to sleep in the chicken coop. When he finally got back into the house, his secret diary entry for the day was, "Why does God hate me?"

This is an incredibly painful story of suffering, so let's step back from Jesse's experience for a moment and talk about how our stress-response systems help us during this kind of ongoing trauma. We've already mentioned the fight-or-flight response. The term was coined in 1915 by the pioneering stress researcher Walter B. Cannon. He used the phrase to describe the acute stress response to a perceived threat, and the physiological changes that go along with it. We will call this the arousal response.

In the arousal response, as we noted earlier, the brain will focus on the threat, tuning out any nonessential input from the body and the outside world. To prepare for fight or flight, our heart rate increases; adrenaline and related stress hormones like cortisol are released, as is sugar stored in our muscles; blood is diverted to our muscles. The general focus of the response is external.

Almost everyone has experienced some version of this activating response when feeling threatened, whether the threat is a visit to the dentist, a fender bender, an impending test, a heated argument, or the prospect of public speaking. You may feel your palms sweat, your heart race; you feel anxious or nervous. This is all due to the activation of the arousal response.

Of course, if you are typical of most people, you don't go from calm to fight in a few seconds (see Figures 5 and 6). When we encounter a potential threat, our initial default behavior is to flock.

*Oprah*: Wait. Please explain *flock*.

*Dr. Perry*: Remember that we humans are very social creatures. We are contagious to the emotions of others; we are continually scanning the relational environment for signs of approval and belonging—as you put it, "How did I do?"

So when there is an unexpected, confusing, or potentially threatening signal, we look to others to help determine what's going on. We look to other people—especially to their facial expressions—for emotional clues about how to interpret the situation. Think of the "Did you just hear that?" or "Did he really just say that?" look you and Gayle might share when you hear something outrageous or inappropriate.

If there is no other person present, or if you get confirmation that this is a threatening situation, you move past flock and scan the environment to put the potential threat in better context.

Next, you might freeze. Picture a dark parking lot. You hear a strange noise, so you stop. Pause. There's a momentary vapor lock in your thinking. This kind of freeze can also happen when you're in a tense interaction where there are conflicting opinions. You may feel like you're not part of the argument, but then someone asks, "So, what's *your* opinion? What should we do?" Before you're able to process and respond, you may simply stare, frozen. And often your response may not feel very "smart"; remember, the more threatened or stressed we are, the less access we have to the smart part of our brain, the cortex (see Figure 6).

As you feel more threatened, you finally get to a fight-or-flee state. To put the entire arousal-response continuum in a nutshell, think of what happens when you come upon a deer in the woods. Deer are hypervigilant, continually flocking. If they hear something or if the behavior of another deer changes, they freeze. This helps them localize the potential threat and makes it harder for sight-based predators to see them. If the threat continues, they flee. But if you cornered the deer, it would fight. Flock, Freeze, Flight, Fight (see Figure 6).

So back to Jesse. During his time in this foster home, his dominant stress response was an arousal response. And he was resisting and running away—fleeing. And ultimately fighting.

One of this family's favorite methods of making the children easier to control was to exhaust them. Forced exercise was routine—in particular, making them run up and down a flight of stairs. One day Jesse finally had enough. When he got to the top of the stairs, he refused to keep going. The foster father raged at him, but Jesse would not budge. A fight ensued. Jesse fell, or was thrown, down the stairs. He sustained the serious head injury that led to his coma and hospitalization.

As we've discussed, our brain uses a couple of key strategies to help us make sense of the world. First, it makes associations between patterns of sensory input that co-occur, creating "memories" from our experiences. Second, it uses these stored memories to categorize and interpret new experience. And if new input is similar enough to previous experience, it will categorize the new experience as similar or equal to the past experience.

Jesse had two sets of trauma memories: one from his abuse as a very young child, the other from his abuse in the foster home. When he was a small child being abused, a fight-or-flight response—resisting, crying, kicking, trying to fight—would simply not have been adaptive; on the contrary, it would have led to more pain and injury. Fortunately, as we mentioned earlier, our brain has a very different stress response to rely on: the dissociative response.

Dissociation is a complex mental capability that we use in everyday life; it involves disengaging from the external world and focusing on our inner world. When we daydream, when we allow our minds to wander, that's a form of dissociation. And like the arousal response, the dissociative response is a continuum. With increasing stress or threat, the dissociative response takes a person deeper and deeper into a protective mode.

Whereas the physiology of the arousal response is to optimize fight or flight, the physiology of dissociation is to help us rest, replenish, survive injury, and tolerate pain. Where arousal increases heart rate, dissociation decreases it. Where arousal sends blood to the muscles, dissociation keeps blood in the trunk, to minimize blood loss in case of injury. Arousal releases adrenaline; dissociation releases the body's own pain killers, enkephalins and endorphins. And dissociation was the only adaptive option available to four-year-old Jesse in abusive moments—the ability to emotionally flee to his inner world.

As part of my assessment when Jesse was in a coma, I was able to obtain unwashed clothing from his biological father and foster father. Despite being unconscious, Jesse had a notable physiological response when reexposed to the scent of these two men. When I placed clothing from the foster father under his nose, he started to thrash and moan, and his heart rate rose from 90 bpm to 162; this profound arousal response was, I believe, due to a set of trauma-related memories from his abuse at the hands of his foster father. (As with Mr. Roseman from Chapter 1, these memories are stored in lower areas of the brain.) When I put clothing from his biological father under his nose, he also reacted—with much less movement and his heart rate initially increasing, then plummeting below 60 bpm. This was consistent with a dissociative response, elicited by activation of the memory of abuse at the hands of his father. Even when the cortex was unavailable (in other words, asleep or in a coma), these evocative cues triggered complex behaviors, emotions, and physiological responses because they are due to memory stored in lower systems in the brain.

The point we're getting at here is that our specific trauma-related responses will depend upon the stress response that was dominant in any given experience. It is possible for one person to have multiple evocative cues that elicit very different behavioral responses. Some trauma-related cues can make you avoidant and shut down; others can enrage and activate. The complex fingerprint of a traumatic experience will be unique for each person. The timing, nature, pattern, and intensity of a traumatic experience can all influence how a person will be impacted.

For Jesse, the story continued. He came out of his coma but unfortunately suffered residual effects. He ultimately went to a retirement home where he lived and worked as a transportation aide. The process of his recovery has much to tell us about the healing power of connection. When we talk about healing and recovery we'll revisit Jesse; for now, know that his story shows the remarkable malleability of the brain, and the power of hope.

Oprah: I think that is what people who read this book are looking for most, the hope that no matter what happened, there is a sliver of light that might lead them forward. The stories you're sharing are what help people realize they are not alone in their trauma. With that in mind, can we talk about trauma and fear for a moment? I know so many people who suffered abuse as a child and seem to live in a constant state of fear, despite the threat no longer being there. Can you explain what happens to the brain when you grow up in fear?

*Dr. Perry*: Yes. A key part of understanding children like Jesse is just that point: They are always in a state of fear. A person will think, learn, feel, and behave differently when they are afraid compared to when they feel safe.

All functioning of the brain is "state-dependent." At any given moment, the collective status of our body's systems and the mind's attention determines the state we're in—and our state can change very quickly. The two biggest categories of state are awake or asleep.

In sleep, there are different stages (for instance, REM, or rapid eye movement, sleep). The same is true of wakefulness; we have different "stages" or states of arousal when awake. We can explore these stages in Figure 6. There's a lot of information here, and some of it we won't get to until later in the book, so let me walk you through it.

Let's start on the left-hand side, with the "Calm" column. In this state we can be calm, relaxed, and let our mind wander and drift; we have access to the smartest part of our brain, the cortex. The next column, "Alert," is where we focus on some aspect of the external world—a conversation, for instance. When we are well-regulated, in balance, we are able to stay in the active alert and calm states for most of our day.

On occasion we will be challenged, surprised, or threatened and will move to the "Alarm" state. When this happens, we start to think in more emotional ways as lower systems in the brain begin to dominate our functioning. Our conversations regress into arguments; the logic of our arguments erodes into emotional or personalized attacks. We act less mature; we often say or do things that we regret.

If we are truly faced with threat, we will progress to the "Fear" state. Here, even lower parts of our brain dominate our functioning. Our problem-solving skills deteriorate; we focus on the moment. And

Figure 6

## STATE-DEPENDENT FUNCTIONING

| *"STATE"* | **CALM** | **ALERT** |
|---|---|---|
| *DOMINANT BRAIN AREAS* | Cortex (DMN) | Cortex (Limbic) |
| *ADAPTIVE "Option" Arousal* | Reflect (create) | Flock (hypervigilance) |
| *ADAPTIVE "Option" Dissociation* | Reflect (daydream) | Avoid |
| *COGNITION* | Abstract (creative) | Concrete (routine) |
| *FUNCTIONAL IQ* | 120–100 | 110–90 |

All functioning of the brain depends on the state we're in. As we move from one internal state to another, there will be a shift in the parts of the brain that are in "control" (dominant); when you are calm, for example, you are able to use the "smartest" parts of your brain (the cortex) to reflect and create. When you feel threatened, those cortical systems become less dominant, and more reactive parts of your brain begin to take over. This continuum goes from calm to terror.

State-dependent shifts result in corresponding changes in a host of brain-mediated functions, including problem-solving capacity, style of thinking (or cognition), and the sphere of concern. In general, the more threatened someone feels, the

| ALARM | FEAR | TERROR |
|---|---|---|
| Limbic<br>(Diencephalon) | Diencephalon<br>(Brainstem) | Brainstem |
| Freeze<br>(resistance) | Flight<br>(defiance) | Fight |
| Comply | Dissociate<br>(paralysis/catatonia) | Faint<br>(collapse) |
| Emotional | Reactive | Reflexive |
| 100–80 | 90–70 | 80–60 |

more control of functioning shifts from higher systems (cortex) to lower systems (diencephalon and brainstem). Fear shuts down many cortical systems.

Adaptive behaviors seen during state-dependent shifts in functioning will differ depending upon which of the two major adaptive response patterns (Arousal and Dissociation) are dominant for any given individual during a stressful or traumatic event.

Default Mode Network (DMN) is a term for a widely distributed network, mostly in the cortex, that is active when an individual is thinking about others, thinking about themselves, remembering the past, and planning for the future.

*in* the moment, of course, this is adaptive. The problems come when individuals get stuck in this state. This is what a pattern of extreme, prolonged stress can do. Think about Jesse. The unpredictability was continuous; the pain, threat, and fear were uncontrollable and, at times, extreme. His stress-response systems adapted—and became sensitized. Jesse was stuck in a permanent state of fear.

Now, as we've suggested before, what is adaptive for children living in chaotic, violent, trauma-permeated environments becomes maladaptive in other environments—especially school. The hyper-vigilance of the Alert state is mistaken for ADHD; the resistance and defiance of Alarm and Fear get labeled as oppositional defiant disorder; flight behavior gets them suspended from school; fight behavior gets them charged with assault. The pervasive misunder-standing of trauma-related behavior has a profound effect on our educational, mental health, and juvenile justice systems.

*Oprah*: And this is why we need *trauma-informed* systems. And why we need to move away from "What is wrong with you?" to "What happened to you?"

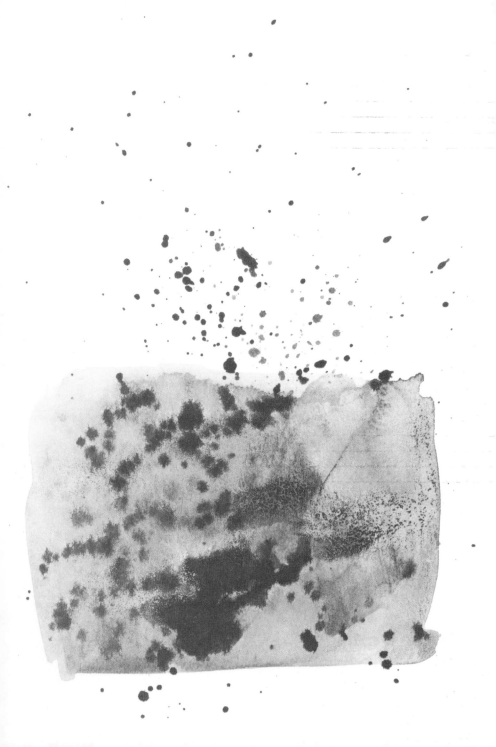

# CHAPTER 4

# THE SPECTRUM OF TRAUMA

*"She wore gray like rain clouds."*

*Those six words, heavy with truth, were what immediately drew me into Cynthia Bond's bestselling novel* Ruby. *In writing the harrowing story of a courageous girl born of tragedy, locked in a battle with the horror she endured and the personal demons she faced, Cynthia drew on her years of working with homeless and at-risk youth—and on her own experience as the survivor of sexual abuse.*

*After joining me for a Book Club conversation, Cynthia wrote an essay for* O Magazine *detailing her mental health struggles. For the longest time, she wrote, she didn't know what was wrong; all she knew was that she viewed the world through a "prism of pain."*

*"For many years," Cynthia wrote, "I rarely slept, kept nightly vigils against my memories. Some mornings it felt like I was weighted to the bed. A deep shame descended: Why couldn't I 'buck up,' 'get over it'? I watched people bounce back from breakups, recover from job loss, foreclosures, and worse. I couldn't fix myself. I began to feel there was something wrong with my character."*

*Cynthia prayed for what she called "the ache" to go away. And like so many people, women in particular, she learned to endure, soldiering on, wearing a mask of strength. Yet in her darkest moments, she contemplated taking her own life.*

*Eventually, she was diagnosed with depression and PTSD. In the wake of the diagnosis, not everyone in her life was supportive. "My voice became suspect. My decisions, my career, my ability to parent were questioned. Some never saw me the same way again." But over time, Cynthia found the support she needed. "I learned . . . that I could have feelings without being disabled by them. That I had done nothing wrong. That I had no reason for shame."*

*Cynthia's story makes me appreciate once more how daunting it can be to deal with past trauma. Many people, when they begin to think about trauma as it applies to their own life, have trouble recognizing the relationship between their early experiences and adult* decision patterns. They rationalize their behavior as "that's just the way it is." Or, in an effort to move quickly past any discomfort they encounter, they make light of it, find ways (both healthy and unhealthy) to soothe it or simply bury it. Trauma is difficult to reconcile.

In its essence, trauma is the lasting effects of emotional shock. If left unexamined, it can have long-term physical, emotional, and social consequences. I've spent my adult life listening to and absorbing stories of those consequences—the havoc wreaked by unresolved trauma.

For me, there are actually two lenses through which to view "what happened to you." There is the science-based explanation of the effect early trauma has on the brain. And then there are the myriad daily actions each of us take throughout our lives that are the result of, and that reflect back on, such trauma. These are the actions that, on the surface, look like poor decisions, bad habits, self-sabotage, self-destruction—the actions that cause other people to judge.

This is why I believe so strongly in the "What happened to you?" approach; it avoids the judgment of "What's wrong with you?"

Addiction of any kind, anxiety, depression, rage, difficulty holding a job, or a cycle of unhealthy relationships: What I know for sure is that all pain is the same. And I believe the despair that runs through nearly all destructive behavior is a deeply rooted feeling of unworthiness. There is a difference between thinking you deserve to be happy and knowing you are worthy of happiness. So often we block our blessings because we don't, at our core, feel that we're enough. Even if you've accumulated a house full of nice things and the picture of your life fits inside a beautiful frame, if you have experienced trauma but haven't excavated it, the wounded parts of you will affect everything you've managed to build.

This chapter is meant to help you recognize the clues indicating that you may have experienced trauma. My hope is that, using the *tools developed by experts like Dr. Perry, you will start to pinpoint the moments that contributed to the person you are today.*

*As you revisit your past, know that no matter what happened, your simply being here, alive, makes you worthy. And know that there is hope. As Cynthia wrote, "Wellness is possible. It happens one moment, one step, at a time."*

*—Oprah*

*Oprah*: You and I have been talking about trauma for over thirty years. At one point, you told me that nearly 40 percent of children under the age of eighteen have suffered some sort of trauma. That is a staggering number.

*Dr. Perry*: Unfortunately, it turns out I was wrong; it's since become clear that the numbers are even worse. A recent study by the National Survey of Children's Health found that almost 50 percent of the children in the United States have had at least one significant traumatic experience. Even more recently, a study from 2019 by the U.S. Centers for Disease Control and Prevention (CDC) found that 60 percent of American adults report having had at least one adverse childhood experience (ACE), and almost a quarter reported three or more ACEs. These numbers are even more sobering when you consider that the CDC researchers believe them to be an underestimate.

*Oprah*: Let's break down what you mean when you use the word *trauma*. Even though it's a word we hear a lot, many people still don't have a clear understanding of its true definition. Is an adverse childhood experience the same as trauma?

*Dr. Perry*: You've homed in on a really important and challenging issue for all of us who study these things. As you suggest, trauma is a word used very casually these days. For most people it means a really bad event or experience, usually one that "sticks," that you don't forget, and that can have an enduring impact on you.

We have always known that people can be changed by the death and carnage seen in combat. For centuries, keen observers of human behavior have described significant emotional and behavioral problems in the wake of war. In 800 BC, in the *Iliad*, Homer described the trauma-related emotional deterioration of Ajax. Four hundred years later, the Greek historian Herodotus described trauma-like symptoms, including hysterical blindness and emotional fatigue, in warriors following the battle of Marathon. Trauma-related mental health effects were known as the "irritable heart" after the American Civil War and "shell shock" following combat in World War I.

Our literature and films are full of "trauma" stories; almost all of the superhero origin stories involve traumatic loss, for example. I'm sure Cynthia Bond's novel *Ruby* isn't the only Oprah's Book Club selection with trauma as a core narrative element; in fact, I'd bet that 80 percent of the selections do. *East of Eden*, for example, is a master class on transgenerational trauma.

Yet trauma has been hard for the academic world to define and therefore understand in its full scope. Part of the challenge is that "bad event" is subjective.

Let's take an example. Consider, say, a fire at an elementary school. A veteran firefighter can walk right up to the flames and put them out, business as usual. In contrast, a first-grader witnessing his classroom burst into flames will experience minutes of intense fear, confusion, and helplessness. This illustrates one of the key issues in understanding a potentially traumatic event: How does the *individual* experience the event? What is going on inside the person; is the stress response activated in extreme or prolonged ways?

*Oprah*: In other words, because the internal experience of a given event varies from person to person, so does the long-term impact.

*Dr. Perry*: Exactly. Any long-term effects are related to several factors, including the nature of your stress response (for example, arousal versus dissociation versus a combination of the two), as well as the intensity and pattern of that response.

Imagine that while the first-grader reacted to the fire in his classroom with terror, a fifth-grader in a different part of the building didn't feel as threatened. To him, the fire was almost exciting; because he was further from the direct threat, he felt safe the entire time.

So we have three people in the same event, each experiencing it differently. And because each experienced it differently, each had a different stress response. Based on her years of experience and practice, the firefighter had a moderate activation of her stress-response systems; the event felt predictable and controllable. For her, it was a resilience-building experience, not a trauma.

For the fifth-grader, there was a temporary activation of his stress response. In a week or so, the acute effects of this activation are gone; he's back to his baseline, "in balance," not traumatized. For the first-grader, however, his stress-response systems were highly activated; he will develop a sensitized stress-response system (see Figures 3 and 5).

*Oprah*: So do we say the fire was a trauma?

*Dr. Perry*: For the first-grader, yes, but not for the fifth-grader. The fifth-grader had an "acute stress reaction," and within weeks returned to his baseline. And for the firefighter, as we said, it was a resilience-building experience.

This is the challenge of studying "traumatic stress." How can we study the impact of trauma if we can't come up with a more standard definition?

In response to this challenge, the Substance Abuse and Mental Health Services Administration (SAMHSA) convened a group of academics and clinicians. They came up with the "three E's" definition of trauma, which articulates what we just talked about: that a trauma has three key aspects—the event, the experience, and the effects. The complexities of these three interrelated components are what should be considered in clinical work and studied in research.

Not very simple or satisfying, I know. The dilemma of defining trauma is not completely solved, and that leads to continued confusing use of the term.

As you and I speak, for example, we are in the middle of a global pandemic, and some have written that it is traumatic that a senior in high school or college doesn't get to have his graduation ceremony. Or that wearing a mask at school will traumatize a child. Or that the pandemic is a trauma for everyone.

Others, like me, have said hold on, these things may be inconvenient and difficult and even tragic, but they aren't necessarily traumatic, and they're certainly not traumatic for everyone. A pandemic is in many ways a shared event, but it is a unique experience for each of us. Many of us will not get sick, lose a job, become homeless, or experience the death of family members or friends. The privilege of some, like me, will be unmasked, while the vulnerability of others will be exposed. The inequities and flaws in our public systems will be magnified. Those with the least will be the most likely to be traumatized. But for many, the experience, while stressful, will not be traumatic.

For me, understanding trauma has always been linked to studying event-specific changes in the stress-response systems. These events can be major and obvious to all, as in the case of physical abuse by a parent. But I believe trauma can also arise from quieter, less obvious experiences, such as humiliation or shaming or other emotional abuse by parents, or the marginalization of a minority child in a majority community (growing up with "out-group" experiences can sensitize the stress-response systems [see Figure 3]). These can result in long-term post-traumatic effects in the brain and the rest of the body.

The specific effects on your health will be determined by a variety of other factors, including genetic vulnerability, the developmental stage at which the traumatic events occurred, history of your previous trauma, your family's history of trauma, and the buffering capacity of healthy relationships, family, and community. But understanding how patterns of stress can influence regulation, or balance, is the key to understanding how *what happened to you* is connected to your health—in all domains, mental, physical, and social.

It has been estimated that childhood adversity plays a major role in 45 percent of all childhood mental health disorders and 30 percent of mental health disorders among adults. These estimates are consistent with other studies that show increased risk for major depression, anxiety, schizophrenia, and other psychotic disorders following childhood trauma or adverse childhood experiences.

*Oprah*: Let's talk more about adverse childhood experiences, or ACEs, as you call them. Walk me through exactly what an ACE is and how the ACE study has helped us better understand the impact of trauma on health.

*Dr. Perry*: The original Adverse Childhood Experience study was published in 1998. The authors created a simple ten-item questionnaire of "adversities" that may have taken place during the first eighteen years of life (see Figure 7). In the original study, seventeen thousand adults filled out the questionnaire to obtain an ACE score ranging from 0 to 10. The authors then looked at the physical, mental, and social health of these adults.

The first ACE epidemiological study found a correlation between the ACE score and the nine major causes of death in adult life. Meaning, the more adversity you had in childhood, the greater your risk for health problems. Subsequent studies using the same data demonstrated similar correlations between an adult ACE score and risk for suicide, mental health problems, substance use and dependence, and a host of other problems.

These ACE studies are some of the most important epidemiology studies done in our lifetime. They have been replicated multiple times. Initially, the study was all but ignored by the medical community and general public. In the last ten years, though, it has become well-known; however, it has been widely misunderstood.

*Oprah*: In what ways?

*Dr. Perry*: There was originally a bit of a pushback due to the design of the study. Because the questionnaire was given to a predominantly white, middle-class sample, people challenged the applicability of the findings to other demographic groups. Another issue was that the ACE questionnaire included only ten adversities—and it left out a host of other potentially traumatic experiences.

The primary misunderstanding of the study, however, is that people confuse correlation with causation. Simply having a high ACE score doesn't mean you *will* get heart disease; it merely means your risk for heart disease goes up.

*Oprah*: I can see how that could be misinterpreted.

*Dr. Perry*: Not every tall person is a good basketball player; and not all good basketball players are tall. But overall, a group of six-foot-five athletes is likely to be better at college basketball than a group of five-foot-five athletes. In the same way, having an ACE score of 5 merely means you will *likely* struggle more than someone with an ACE score of 1.

Let's keep thinking this through. If you go to a college campus and find all the six-foot-five students, only a few of them will be on the varsity basketball team. Many of them will be uncoordinated and nonathletic. It's the same with the ACE score. Many people with ACE scores of 5 are healthy, productive, positive, and

*Figure 7*

# ADVERSE CHILDHOOD EXPERIENCE SURVEY

Prior to your eighteenth birthday...

1. Did a parent or other adult in the household often or very often . . . Swear at you, insult you, put you down, or humiliate you? Or act in a way that made you afraid that you might be physically hurt?

    **No_____ If Yes, enter 1 _____**

2. Did a parent or other adult in the household often or very often . . . Push, grab, slap, or throw something at you? Or ever hit you so hard that you had marks or were injured?

    **No_____ If Yes, enter 1 _____**

3. Did an adult or person at least five years older than you ever . . . Touch or fondle you or have you touch their body in a sexual way? Or attempt or actually have oral, anal, or vaginal intercourse with you?

    **No_____ If Yes, enter 1 _____**

4. Did you often or very often feel that . . . No one in your family loved you or thought you were important or special? Or your family didn't look out for each other, feel close to each other, or support each other?

    **No_____ If Yes, enter 1 _____**

5. Did you often or very often feel that . . . You didn't have enough to eat, had to wear dirty clothes, and had no one to protect you? Or your parents were too drunk or high to take care of you or take you to the doctor if you needed it?

    **No_____ If Yes, enter 1 _____**

6. Were your parents ever separated or divorced?

**No_____ If Yes, enter 1 _____**

7. Was your mother or stepmother . . . Often or very often pushed, grabbed, slapped, or had something thrown at her? Or sometimes, often, or very often kicked, bitten, hit with a fist, or hit with something hard? Or ever repeatedly hit over at least a few minutes or threatened with a gun or knife?

**No_____ If Yes, enter 1 _____**

8. Did you live with anyone who was a problem drinker or alcoholic, or who used street drugs?

**No_____ If Yes, enter 1 _____**

9. Was a household member depressed or mentally ill, or did a household member attempt suicide?

**No_____ If Yes, enter 1 _____**

10. Did a household member go to prison?

**No_____ If Yes, enter 1 _____**

Now add up your "Yes" answers: _____ This is your ACE score.

don't struggle. And some people with an ACE score of 1 will have major problems.

Again, the ACE studies are *tremendously* important. But the ACE score doesn't have much real predictive power on an individual basis, or as a clinical tool. It's only a very superficial glance at "what happened to you"—not the deep and prolonged exploration required to truly understand our personal journey. Think about how superficial, and bizarre, your interviews would be if you merely handed out a form with ten questions and got a single number from each guest. The ACE score doesn't tell their story; the number can't *be* their story.

What the ACE score does not tell you is the timing, pattern, and intensity of stress and distress or the presence of buffering or healing factors. It leaves out some of the most important variables involved in predicting health and risk.

Let me give you two examples from our work. Over the years, we have collected developmental data from over seventy thousand individual cases in twenty-five countries. This includes young children, children, youth, and adults. We've taken detailed histories of trauma and adversity as well as histories of "relational health" (essentially, connectedness—i.e., the nature, quality, and quantity of connection to family, community, and culture).

Our major finding is that your history of relational health—your connectedness to family, community, and culture—is more predictive of your mental health than your history of adversity (see Figure 8). This is similar to the findings of other researchers looking at the power of positive relationships on health. Connectedness has the power to counterbalance adversity.

Our second major finding is that the *timing* of adversity makes a huge difference in determining overall risk. Put simply, if you experience trauma at age two, it will have more impact on your health than the same trauma taking place at age seventeen. Unfortunately, the ACE survey does not help you make that distinction; it asks only whether any of those ten adversities were present during the first eighteen years of your life.

When we look a little deeper into the timing of developmental risk, a powerful observation emerges. The basic finding is that the experiences of the first two months of life have a disproportionately important impact on your long-term health and development. This has to do with the remarkably rapid growth of the brain early in life, and the organization of those all-important core regulatory networks (see Figure 2).

If, in the first two months of life, a child experienced high adversity with minimal relational buffering but was then put into a healthier environment for the next twelve years, their outcomes were worse than the outcomes of children who had low adversity and healthy relational connection in the first two months but then spent the next twelve years with high adversity.

Think of that: The child who has only two months of really bad experiences does worse than the child with almost twelve years of bad experiences, all because of the timing of the experiences.

This sounds discouraging. But we believe that poor outcomes are not inevitable; in fact, we believe that this is a perfect example of why we need developmentally informed, trauma-aware systems.

Think back to our earlier conversations about how important attentive, responsive caregiving is in providing the organizing experiences for the infant's stress-response systems. Remember that if the life experiences of the first two months include inconsistent or unpredictable stress, this pattern of activation creates a sensitized stress response (see Figures 3 and 5). That leads to a cascade of problems—trauma-related problems. And even when these children are no longer in high-risk settings, their problems have to be addressed by caregivers, pediatricians, menta health providers, and educators. But if these people misunderstand what's going on, if these systems focus on "What is wrong with you?"—as, unfortunately, they typically do—the children

## Figure 8

# THE IMPACT OF DEVELOPMENTAL EXPERIENCE

## THE BALANCE BETWEEN ADVERSITY AND CONNECTEDNESS

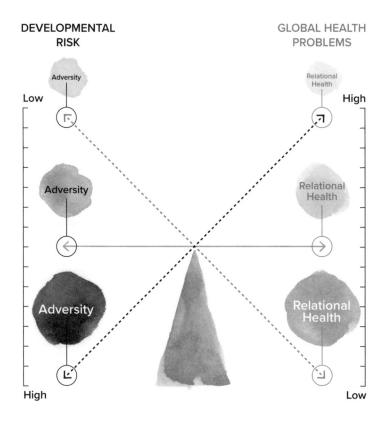

With high connectedness and low adversity during development (blue dashed line), the balance of developmental risk is tipped in the direction of lower risk for mental, social, and physical health problems. In contrast, high adversity and minimal connectedness (black dashed line) increases developmental risk and the probability of significant problems in overall health.

won't get better. They will continue to struggle. Their emotional reactivity and behavior problems will be viewed without a developmental or trauma lens, which could lead to ineffective interventions.

We believe these children could live happier, healthier lives if the homes, schools, health-care, and mental health systems they grew up in replaced "What is wrong with you?" with "What happened to you?"

And we recognize the power and potential of very early childhood. Think of the impact just a few months of consistent, predictable support for a young parent could make. For the child, it could create a positive jump start in life that would lead to the development of more resilient stress-response systems. And in turn, these regulated stress-response systems would help ensure healthy development in higher parts of the brain.

*Oprah*: This makes it clear how important prevention is. If we could support young parents in those first months, it would be like giving their children resilience-building megavitamins.

*Dr. Perry*: And for me, the really fascinating part is the power of brief but positive caregiving interactions. Some of the children we studied had attentive and responsive care for only the first two months of life—and then their world imploded. Years of chaos, threat, instability, and trauma followed those positive first two months—yet they did much better than children who experienced initial trauma and neglect followed by years of attentive, supportive care. It is the timing that is so important. The value of early intervention programs, even those that have only brief "doses" of positive interaction, can't be underestimated.

*Oprah*: The timing is crucial. But what happens if you don't get what you need early on? Can you make it up? Can you heal from trauma?

*Dr. Perry*: Of course. That is the good news, which we will explore much more in later chapters. For now, though, this issue of time and timing is so important. The neural networks involved in relational connection and regulation are very responsive to *moments*. This means that a meaningful dose of therapeutic interaction isn't forty-five minutes once a week. When you're dealing with an intense trauma, we've found that the "tolerable" dose is only seconds long.

*Oprah*: Really?

*Dr. Perry*: You can stand the emotional intensity of visiting the wreckage of your trauma-fractured life for only a few seconds before your brain starts to do things to protect you from the pain. I saw this behavior in a three-year-old boy I worked with some time ago.

This boy was sitting with his mother when there was a home invasion, and he witnessed his mother being killed. We started working with both the boy and his father right afterward. After about six weeks, I received a call from the father. "My son is suicidal," he said. "He just tried to kill himself."

Now, it's very rare for three-year-olds to try to kill themselves. But I asked the father to tell me what happened. He said, "He ran into traffic after we were talking about missing Mom." I asked him to explain *exactly* what happened. He told me they'd been in the grocery store and the son had been sitting in the cart while they were checking out. The boy looked at the checkout clerk and said, "My mom's dead. She got killed."

The clerk said, "Oh, honey, I'm sorry." And that was it. But the father was worried that the boy needed to say more. He thought, *We've got to get it out. We've got to get to the trauma.* And so, as they're walking to the parking lot, he asked his son, "Are you thinking about Mom?"

The boy didn't answer. His father continued, "You know, I miss Mom, and it's okay to talk about it."

The father spoke gently, reminding the boy of loving times with his mother, but "revisiting" these emotional moments was not controlled by the boy. It was overwhelming. As the father talked, the little boy started to rock himself, then moan, then cover his ears, then rock frantically—all in an effort to regulate himself.

The father tried to comfort him with words. "It's okay to talk about Mom." But the boy jumped out of the cart and, as the father said, began to run around the parking lot.

This behavior reflects a predictable sequence when the arousal response is activated. As the arousal systems activate, they shut down the top part of the brain (see Figure 6), and the lower, primitive parts of the brain take over. The thinking part of this poor little boy's brain was shut down. He wasn't planning to kill himself; he wasn't *planning* anything. He was simply trying to "flee"—to get away from the painful images of his mother's murder, which his father was evoking by his probing questioning.

The father had good intentions, but it wasn't the right dose for a therapeutic moment. So, back to the issue of time. When the little boy looks up at the clerk and sees a woman about the age of his mother, with the same hair color, it's an evocative cue. For a moment he is back to the memory of Mom, the murder. He looks at the clerk, makes one brief comment—five seconds, tops—and gets reassurance. That was enough. One little fragment in the wreckage—a dose of therapeutic revisiting that he controlled. Because it is through controllable, brief revisits that the sensitized system can slowly, painfully be "reset." Ideally, thousands of such therapeutic moments can be provided by the therapeutic web of loving, sensitive people in your life.

Think about how you've handled difficulty in your own life. With things that are very hard to deal with, you don't want to talk about the pain or loss or fear for forty-five minutes nonstop. You want to talk with a really good friend for maybe two or three minutes about some aspect of it. When it gets too painful, you step back, you want to be distracted. And maybe you want to talk more later on. It is the therapeutic dosing that really leads to healing. Moments. Fully present, powerful but brief.

*Oprah*: What you're saying makes me so grateful for my relationship with Gayle King. She has been a constant in my life since we met, way back in 1976, when we were both working at a Baltimore news station. Even though we now live on different coasts, in different time zones, and lead very busy lives, we talk every day. I have been her therapist. She has been my therapist. I've never been to an actual therapist, but I think our relationship, as we run through everything that's happening and switch back and forth between what's on my mind and what's on hers—I think we are actually dosing.

*Dr. Perry*: You back off and then circle back.

*Oprah*: Right, you laugh about something else and that triggers something new. Then maybe you go back to the difficult experience or not. It's just what happens when you're talking to your girlfriends all the time.

*Dr. Perry*: That's right. That is healing. That is the essence of a therapeutic experience.

*Oprah*: You end up feeling better because you've released it. You've gotten reinforced, just as the little boy was "heard" and reassured by the clerk.

*Dr. Perry*: Yes! You've had that positive human interaction that's nurturing. It is rewarding, regulating, and bonding.

*Oprah*: I've just had an *Aha!* What you're really looking for is somebody to reinforce the idea that *Hey, I'm not crazy. I'm thinking or feeling this way because of something that happened to me, and I'm having a reasonable reaction.* And that person validates that for you.

*Dr. Perry*: Exactly, and, in "seeing" you, they regulate you. And for this little boy, over the years, thousands upon thousands of little positive interactions with Dad, grandparents, neighbors, friends, and teachers provided the rewarding, regulating, and healing experiences that helped him. Today he is a healthy, positive young man. The loss of his mother can still bring sadness and longing, but it passes. At baseline he is open, curious, and kind; he is not dysregulated or sad or impaired. The formal aspects of therapy lasted about a year. It was these other therapeutic moments, taking place every day for twenty years, that really helped him rebuild a healthy inner world from the trauma-shattered wreckage of his three-year-old self.

*Oprah*: Did this little boy have PTSD? So many of us learned about PTSD in context of combat veterans, like Mr. Roseman in Chapter 1. But I know trauma at any age can cause PTSD, correct?

*Dr. Perry*: Yes, trauma at any age can cause a cluster of symptoms we call post-traumatic stress disorder (PTSD). And this boy did have PTSD. If you remember those three "components" of trauma, the three E's—the event, the experience, and the effects—PTSD is about the effects. It's a specific syndrome—or collection of symptoms—that can occur in the wake of a traumatic event or events, and it's one of the mental disorders in the *Diagnostic and Statistical Manual* (DSM), which is the guide most clinicians use to classify mental health problems.

A person diagnosed with PTSD has four main symptom clusters following a traumatic event or events. As you mentioned, Mike Roseman, the Korean War veteran who was triggered by the motorcycle backfiring, had PTSD.

The first cluster is "intrusive" symptoms. These include recurring, unwanted images and thoughts of the traumatic event, and dreams or nightmares about it. One way to think about these symptoms is that they're related to the brain's efforts to make sense of the world. Often when a traumatic event takes place, it is so threatening and so far outside our usual experience that it doesn't fit our working model of the world. If you recall our earlier conversations, our mind is always working to preserve the worldview that was created early in our lives. *People are good. Parents are here to protect us. Schools are safe.* The mind wants to see what we believe, so it clings to things that support those beliefs—that worldview—and ignores things that don't. But trauma shatters this inner landscape. Your worldviews are broken to pieces. *People can't be trusted. I'm terrified of my father, he hurts me. School is where my friends were shot.*

Trauma leaves you shipwrecked. You are left to rebuild your inner world. Part of the rebuilding, the healing process, is revisiting the shattered hull of your old worldview; you sift through the wreckage looking for what remains, seeking your broken pieces. Dreams, intrusive images of the trauma, and reenactment play are your mind struggling to make sense of your new reality. As you revisit the shipwreck, piece by piece, you find a fragment and move it to your new, safer place in the now-altered landscape. You build a new worldview. That takes time. And many visits to the wreckage. And this process involves both unconscious and conscious repetitive "reenactment" behaviors, or writing, drawing, sculpting, or playing. Again and again, you revisit the site of the earthquake, look through the wreckage, take something, and move it to a safe haven. That's part of the healing process. I'm simplifying very complex processes, which we'll talk about more when we focus on healing.

The second cluster is "avoidant" symptoms. We believe that these symptoms arise when someone feels distressed after being reexposed to people, places, or other reminders of the original traumatic events. Remember Mr. Roseman saying he hated the Fourth of July? Because he was consciously aware that fireworks were evocative cues, he avoided celebrations that involved them. In some ways, avoidant behaviors are an attempt to regain control over what feels like the uncontrollability of the traumatic experience. You may also recall that avoidance is part of a dissociative response to a threat (see Figure 6). When someone is in an unavoidable, distressing situation, avoidant behaviors can be protective.

A person can also develop avoidant behaviors without making the direct connection to a traumatic cue from the past. This is often true when the abuse or trauma took place within the context of early caregiving relationships. If a child was abused in the context of an intimate relationship (by a parent, for example), they will find intimacy—emotional and physical closeness—threatening. They will often long to be connected but find themselves anxious, confused, or overwhelmed when they get close to someone. They will avoid intimacy in a relationship; if intimacy can't be avoided, they will sabotage or undermine the relationship. This is one of the most common but least appreciated effects of developmental trauma.

*Oprah*: So when you have PTSD, you become triggered in the moment because the "memory" from the trauma is activated. And people's response varies because the PTSD reaction is in direct proportion to how the traumatic event affected you in the first place.

*Dr. Perry*: Remember our earlier discussion of making associations? The traumatic experience creates a set of trauma-related "memories"; these become "connected" to the type of stress response that played out in the specific traumatic event.

You'll recall that Jesse, the boy in the coma, had two very distinct responses to different evocative cues. For Mike Roseman, the evocative cue of the motorcycle backfire activated his arousal response—because the arousal response is what was activated when he was in combat. The sound of gunfire—or a motorcycle backfiring—led to increased heart rate, the instinct to duck and cover, etc.

But in another patient, a sound like gunfire might elicit an entirely different response. I once had a patient, Bisa, a young refugee woman from Somalia who had lived through brutal tribal warfare. She had watched, helpless, while her younger brother was forced to shoot her parents. Much more trauma followed before she made it to Canada. For Bisa, as it had for Mike Roseman, gunfire became an evocative cue. But whereas it provoked an arousal response in Mike, in Bisa it prompted a dissociative shutdown. Her trauma had comprised moments of inescapable, unbearable pain. Her response was to escape inside herself (see Figure 6). Her heart rate decreased. In the extreme, she fainted. Later, when she'd hear a loud, unexpected noise, the association with gunfire would make her collapse; she'd actually lose consciousness.

A colleague of mine, a photojournalist, was present at one of the first refugee camps created to house victims of the Rwandan Civil War. There were people milling around like zombies, expressionless, silent. Just as my colleague was asking why some of them were wearing helmets, gunfire came from the jungle around the camp and several of the people fainted on the spot. They wore helmets so their heads wouldn't be injured when they fell.

*Oprah*: So that was from what you describe as an overactive and overly reactive dissociative response, right?

*Dr. Perry*: Absolutely. Which brings us back to our list of PTSD symptoms. We've discussed the first two symptom clusters, intrusive symptoms and avoidant symptoms, and now we get to the third: changes in mood and thinking. This can include depressive symptoms—sadness, loss of pleasure from anything, a sense of guilt, an overfocus on negative things, and basically a feeling of emotional and physical exhaustion.

Finally, the fourth symptom cluster is an alteration in arousal and reactivity. These are symptoms related to the sensitized stress-response networks being overactive and overly reactive. They include anxiety, hypervigilance, increased startle response, high and variable heart rate, and sleep problems.

When someone has symptoms in each of those four categories, the DSM label is PTSD. It is really important to remember, however, that PTSD is not the only way that trauma impacts our mental and physical health. The adverse effects of trauma that we discussed at the beginning of this chapter can have just as significant an impact on someone's life. In fact, the majority of the long-term effects of trauma don't manifest as PTSD.

*Oprah*: As you're talking, here's what I keep thinking: Depression, anxiety, PTSD—these seem to be the big three when it comes to the long-term mental and emotional effects of trauma. So if we know that there are *fifty million* children who have experienced trauma, that means there are countless millions of adults carrying that hurt through their lives, their jobs, their relationships, and then passing it on to their children. And those adults may not even realize what happened to them.

*Dr. Perry*: Not only do *they* not realize what happened, but their partners, doctors, and work colleagues don't, either. And that leads to so much misunderstanding. And sometimes these misunderstandings have tragic consequences.

We have talked a lot about how the actions of caregivers influence the child, but it's important to remember that those caregivers were also children influenced by *their* caregivers. The effects of trauma stretch far and wide across generations and across communities, and it's important to always come back to our central question with compassion: What happened to you?

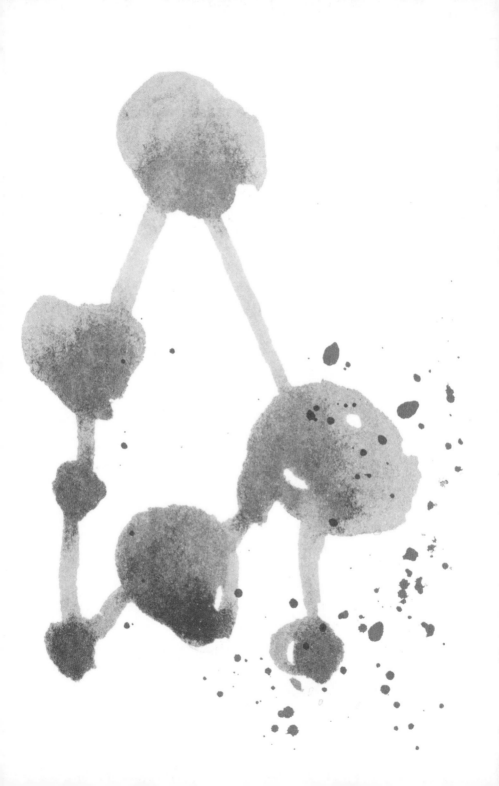

# CHAPTER 5

---

# CONNECTING THE DOTS

*For much of my adult life, being alone at night was extremely stress-*
*ful. Even in Chicago, where I lived on the fifty-seventh floor of a build-*
*ing staffed with security and a doorman, I didn't feel safe. In fact, one*
*night, after living in the condo a few years, I felt so acutely frightened*
*that I convinced myself I had to leave because something bad was*
*going to happen to me if I didn't. I actually got up from bed, left my*
*home, and checked into the hotel next door. I felt safer in the hotel*
*because no one would know I was there. My fears didn't make sense*
*to me, and they were getting worse. I knew I needed to figure out*
*what was going on, but I had no idea where to even begin.*

*At the same time, Chicago was reeling from one of the country's*
*first-ever school shootings. On May 20, 1988, Laurie Dann walked*
*into a second-grade classroom in the North Shore suburb of Win-*
*netka and opened fire. Six children were shot, and eight-year-old*
*Nick Corwin was killed.*

*In the aftermath of the shooting, angry and anguished parents*
*were calling for the school's doors to be locked and chained and*
*manned by security guards. One day I read an article that explained*
*why the school principal refused to implement these changes; he*
*said chaining the doors would send a message to the children that*
*they were unsafe.*

*And all of a sudden, out of the blue, while reading this article, I*
*started to cry.*

*Not just for the children and their families who were picking up*
*the pieces after a tragedy, but because the words of the principal*
*who refused to barricade the children triggered a long-forgotten*
*memory of an event I hadn't thought of in years.*

*Growing up in Mississippi, I always slept with my grandmother. My*
*grandfather, who had dementia, slept in a side room. One night I was*
*suddenly awakened to see my grandfather standing over the bed.*
*Even before I opened my eyes, I could sense my grandmother's fear.*
*I could feel her heightened awareness as she slowly repeated,*

*"Earlest, get back to bed. Earlest, get back to bed." He wouldn't go. He was trying to choke her, fighting to get his hands around her neck. When she finally managed to push him off her and run to the door, she cried out for one of our neighbors we called Cousin Henry, who lived down the road. "Henry! Henry! Henry!" Henry was blind, but without hesitation he came in the middle of the night to help my grandmother put my grandfather back in his bedroom. My grand-mother then wedged a chair under the doorknob of her bedroom door and found some cans to put around the bed. The next morning she tied those cans together and hung them from the door. And, every night for the rest of my days living with my grandmother, the cans were on the door and the chair was up under the knob. I would try to sleep while listening to make sure the cans didn't move.*

*When I read about the principal who would not put chains on the doors, I had an* Aha. *The cans on my grandmother's door sent the very message the principal was trying to avoid sending to his young students. The chains would perhaps have protected the chil-dren, but in the principal's mind, it was more damaging to constantly remind them of a traumatic incident and make them believe they were unsafe.*

*I finally connected the dots as to why I was afraid to be home alone at night. The attack on my grandmother, while we were asleep and at our most vulnerable, had been traumatizing. Obviously it left deep emotional scars. Even as an adult, as I tried to sleep, my mind was conditioned to stay in a constant state of arousal, prepared for attack.*

*Making that connection, finally understanding both the cause and effect of my sleep trouble, was a game changer for me. Though I can still feel myself reacting to the deep stress points born in my grand-mother's bedroom all those years ago, I now have the tools and understanding to step back, observe what I'm feeling, and choose how to move through the fear.*

*As you consider your individual response patterns, know that by putting a small moment of space between the immediate feeling and your instinctive reaction, you are allowing yourself to stay present and ultimately regain control.*

—Oprah

*Oprah:* Is it possible for a heightened sense of fear to be inherited?

*Dr. Perry:* Well, let me expand the question.

*Oprah:* I should have guessed! You're not going to just answer "yes" or "no," are you? You're going to make this more complicated, right?

*Dr. Perry:* Yes. Yes, I am. Because you're getting at "What happened to *us*?"—and that influences who we become in complicated ways. We absorb things from previous generations and pass them on to the next generation. Our genes, family, community, society, and culture are all part of this. So your question about fear being inherited is central to understanding trauma, especially "historical trauma."

Let's use a fear of dogs as an example here. This fear may be based in personal experience—being bitten by a dog as a child, for example. The child's brain created associations between dogs and threat, similar to what happened to Mr. Roseman from his combat experiences. But we know that some people have an intense fear of dogs despite no real personal history with dogs. Where does that come from? I would suggest that this fear may come from transgenerational transmission (see Figure 9). Imagine, for example, growing up in a world where dogs were trained to hunt, track, and attack humans. Slave hounds have been described by Tyler Parry, a leading scholar on colonization and slavery, as the "most effective and terrifying tool for disciplining black bodies and dominating their space." Generations later, dogs were used the same way to intimidate and terrorize civil rights marchers in the South, reinforcing a transgenerational fear of dogs for many. If you remember our conversations about emotional contagion, it is not hard to imagine a child "feeling" fear around a dog when their parent holds their hand harder or hurries to cross the street to avoid someone walking their dog. The fear of the grandparent becomes the fear of the parent, which becomes the fear of the child.

Understanding *what* we "inherit" and *how* we "inherit" is necessary for the insight required to make intentional change—change at the individual level (such as healing after trauma) *and* change at the cultural level (such as identifying and changing destructive policies that embed racism, for example).

*Oprah*: Over the years, I've had conversations with the author and spiritual teacher Iyanla Vanzant about how, in so many ways, we are a product of our ancestors. Iyanla says, "Every family has patterns and pathologies of thought, belief, and behavior that are passed on from one generation to another in the same way that a physical characteristic is passed on." And even though we like to celebrate the strengths and successes of those who came before us, Iyanla says, "Many of these conscious and unconscious characteristics are powerful and productive. Others are not."

So I'm curious to know what the science says. From a biological perspective, can certain psychological traits, emotional characteristics, and behavior patterns be passed down from one family member to another over long spans of time?

*Dr. Perry*: Absolutely—generation after generation. And there are multiple pathways we use to "pass down" these characteristics (see Figure 9). Take your question about fear, for example. Strictly speaking, when you ask if we *inherit* a sense of fear, you're asking if this trait is encoded in our genetics and passed to us from our parents, and the answer to that is a bit fuzzy.

But if we ask a slightly different question—*Is fear transmissible from generation to generation? Can the fearfulness of a parent be transmitted to the child?*—the answer is an emphatic yes.

At our core, as we've said, we are relational beings—social creatures. And because of that, we are neurobiologically tuned in to other people. Part of our brain is continually monitoring others around us.

*Figure 9*

## MECHANISMS OF
## TRANSGENERATIONAL TRANSMISSION

**Genetic**

— DNA

**Epigenetic (modification and control of gene expression)**

— Histone modification

— DNA methylation

**Intrauterine**

— Maternal milieu (e.g., stress)

— Environmental toxins

— Other (e.g., alcohol, drugs)

**Perinatal Experience**

— Bonding and attachment (shaping primary regulatory and relational core)

**Postnatal**

— Family-mediated (e.g., language, values, and beliefs)

**Postnatal**

— Education-, community-, and culture-mediated

We're trying to understand other people's intentions and feelings. This is part of our making sense of the world. We are sensing and absorbing the emotions of those around us. This is particularly true when it comes to the people we spend most time with and are most dependent upon. Children, especially, are very contagious to the emotions of the people around them. Think of you and your grandmother in the story you just shared. You felt fear. Her fear was passed to you—you "caught" her fear and carried it into your generation.

*Oprah*: Yes, I could feel her fear. And she was a strong woman who was in charge of the house; this was an unusual response for her. So I knew that it was a dangerous situation, and I believe it changed me on a cellular level.

When I think about the African American community, I see how trauma can trace back for generations—all the way back to slavery. Hundreds of years of internalizing the trauma of racism, segregation, brutality, fear, and the dismantling of the nuclear family—all of it replicated and repeated over and over at the micro level of the individual and eventually seen and felt at the macro level of society. That's why the Black Lives Matter protests of 2020 were so powerful. The individual at the micro level and society at the macro level had both reached an apex of pain.

*Dr. Perry*: And I would say that if we better understand how this pain—this trauma—is passed from generation to generation, we have a better chance of intentionally and effectively stopping it.

This comes back to *transmissibility*—emotional contagion. The word *transmissible* is used to describe the ability of a trait (or skill, belief, etc.) to be passed on from one person to another. When children raised in a household that speaks only Spanish grow up and speak Spanish, they didn't "inherit" Spanish. The capacity to make associations between sound and image is primarily genetic, but the

*129*

specific ways we turn that genetic capacity into a language are not. There are no genes for Chinese or English or Spanish.

But language *is* transmissible. Early in life, the language-related systems in our brain's cortex are so spongelike that they change when we interact with people in ways that involve speech. By speaking with the baby, we change her brain. This allows her to learn her family's language.

This same experience-dependent process applies to many other traits, as well as to values and beliefs. These are not genetically coded—they are learned, absorbed, sometimes modified, and then taught to the next generation by example, intentional instruction, and inertia. There *are* complex traits, such as altruism, that require genetic superstructure, but how we incorporate that into the complex beliefs and practices of Buddhism or Christianity or Islam is not genetic. There may be genetic elements to being wary or defensive when interacting with someone very different from your family or clan of origin, but racism is a learned set of beliefs about the superiority of a people, and racism in practice is about power, dominance, and oppression.

The language we speak, the beliefs we hold—both good and bad—are passed from generation to generation through experience. And so many aspects of the human experience are invented—as opposed to simply springing up from our genes. Ten thousand years ago, humankind had the genetic potential to read a book, yet not one single human on the planet could read; the genetic potential to play the piano existed, yet not one person could play; the genetic potential to dunk a basketball, type a sentence, ride a bicycle—all that potential existed, but it all remained unexpressed.

Humankind, more than any other species, can take the accumulated, distilled experiences of previous generations and pass these inventions, beliefs, and skills to the next generation. This is sociocultural evolution. We learn from our elders, and we invent, and we pass what we've learned and invented to the next generations. And the organ that allows this is the human brain—specifically, the cortex. As we've said before, the cortex is the most uniquely human part of our body, and, no surprise, it gives rise to the most uniquely human capabilities: speech, language, abstract thinking, reflecting on the past, planning for the future. Our hopes, dreams, and a major part of our worldview are mediated by our cortex.

*Oprah*: So, if generations of experiences that contribute to our worldview are negative, how do we deal with that?

*Dr. Perry*: To start, we need to be aware of the ways in which every aspect of our world can influence us in powerful and often unknown ways.

Our media, our institutions and systems, our communities—all are infused with some elements of bias. In so many instances we pass on the language of superiority, dominance, and oppression in quiet and invisible but powerful ways.

The cortex, which mediates reading, writing, math, history—as well as our beliefs and values—is incredibly malleable. We all know that if you experience repetitive instruction that involves looking at letters, sounding out words, and listening to others read, you will ultimately build your own neurobiological capacity to read. We *learn* to read. By stimulating specific neural networks in patterned, repetitive ways, we change the brain. This is an experience-based transmission of a skill from one generation to the next; teaching a child changes their brain. And with this changed brain, the child can grow up and teach what she has learned to someone in the next generation. There is transgenerational transmission—something is passed on to the next generation.

The same is true of our beliefs—our humane and compassionate beliefs as well as our hateful, oppressive, dehumanizing beliefs. The very same malleability of the brain—the spongelike quality that lets infants absorb and learn the language of their parents—also allows children to absorb the beliefs, good and bad, of influential adults.

So, understanding the way we pass things to the next generation is important. If we want to enrich the transmission of humane, compassionate values, beliefs, and practices, and minimize the transmission of hateful, destructive beliefs, we need to be very mindful of what we're exposing our children to. Are they spending time with people who are different from them? Are they seeing diversity celebrated? Or are they being raised to fear and judge anyone who doesn't think or look or speak like they do? Generational transmission of bias *can* be disrupted. We can stop passing hateful, destructive, and false beliefs to the next generation, but to do so we must be exceedingly intentional about all of the ways we influence our babies, toddlers, and young children. We have to think about the images they see in the magazines we read, the people we welcome into our homes, the ways we treat others who look different from us. And that is just the very beginning; so many aspects of our world need to shift. But all of these things can influence the transgenerational transmission process.

*Oprah*: Which brings me to what I've known innately all my life, and have come to understand more profoundly over time: Everything matters. Everything that's ever happened to you, ever happened to your mother, ever happened to the mother before her, and to the father, and so on—everything matters.

*Dr. Perry*: Your own experiences and the echoes of your ancestors' experiences influence the way you think, feel, and behave. They are major determinants of your health. And being aware of this can help us remember that everything we do right now is going to echo into the future. Our actions matter; we are impacting the next generations. So are we being as mindful as we could?

*Oprah*: Our actions have a tremendous ripple effect—which makes it all the more critical to our evolution that we understand what happened to us.

*Dr. Perry*: And this brings us back to your simple question, "Is it possible for a heightened sense of fear to be inherited?"—so let's go back and finish answering that question.

One of the most important ways we transmit "information" to the next generation is through our genes. And some aspects of our stress-response systems are "heritable"; there are genetic mechanisms that play a role in how our core regulatory networks (CRNs) function (see Figure 2).

Some people appear to have a genetically influenced capacity for "hardiness"—they can tolerate a wider range of sensory complexity and stressors. It takes more to dysregulate these people. In contrast, other people appear to be born with a "sensitive" stress response. They are more easily overwhelmed by minor shifts in sensory complexity. Sometimes these people have what's referred to as a "difficult to soothe" temperament noticeable at birth.

In addition to heritable genetics related to stress regulation, there are also heritable "epigenetic" factors. Epigenetics is another one of those widely used and poorly understood terms in our field, so let me give a very brief overview.

Every cell in your body has the same genes, but not every cell has the same genes "turned on." This is because some genes are specific for bone, some for blood, some for neurons, and so forth. During development, the genes involved in, say, muscle-cell machinery are turned on in muscle cells, while the genes for blood, bone, and brain are turned off. As cells become "specialized," many of their genes are shut off.

However, in some situations, for instance starvation, the body sends chemical messages to the genes that have been turned off, telling them to turn back on. *Hey, we normally don't need you, but since we are starving, we have to use sugar and fats more efficiently, so we're turning you on to do that work.* These are called epigenetic changes—"epi" meaning "above" in Greek, because the actual genes are not changing, but cellular mechanisms "above" the gene can turn key genes on and turn others off. These gene regulatory processes are continually at work in our body, trying to keep us "in balance"— well-regulated and as healthy as we can be.

Now, as we've talked about, different patterns of stress can lead to either sensitization or resilience. In both cases, epigenetic changes are involved in altering the sensitivity of the CRNs. This is another example of the remarkable flexibility of the body to make changes to keep you in balance.

In some cases, these epigenetic changes will be stored in the egg or sperm and passed to the next generation. Go back a few centuries and imagine a young man captured in Africa, brutally enslaved, shackled, starved, transported by slave ship to a life of bondage that will be filled with loss, violence, and multiple forms of trauma. Surviving such extreme, multiple, and ongoing traumas—as millions of remarkable human beings did—would likely create a cascade of adaptive changes all the way down to the regulation of gene expression. To be clear, the genes themselves would not change, rather, they could, as we've discussed, be turned on and off. This young man's children, and grandchildren, still enslaved and enduring other traumas, would benefit from these epigenetic, molecular adaptations. Yet as we've discussed, there is a cost to having a persistently sensitized stress-response network. It is likely that, over the generations, in different environments, once-adaptive changes would become maladaptive.

Picture an infant born with the stress-response apparatus already primed for trauma, ready for an unpredictable, chaotic, and threatening world. If the world is no longer as extremely chaotic, threatening, and unpredictable, the epigenetic changes that prime this infant for chaos may lead to a somewhat distorted process of creating his "worldview." The study of epigenetics is still very young, and there is much more to learn, but it is conceivable that the experiences of our grandparents, great-grandparents, and ancestors even further back have had a significant influence on the way we're going to express our DNA. And—to your original question—a significant influence on our sense of fear.

The good news is that the brain remains changeable. As you might expect, the epigenetic mechanisms that regulate genes are reversible—they wouldn't provide much adaptive advantage if they weren't. Just as threat and trauma can lead to epigenetic changes, so can nurturing interactions reverse those. Environments and challenges change—and, if we are to stay in balance, so must our physiology.

*Oprah*: We talked earlier about how childhood adversity can impact us. And now we've talked about how emotional and behavioral patterns and experiences and beliefs can be passed down from prior generations. It clarifies for me on such a deeper level that understanding "what happened" to someone as opposed to "what's wrong" with them should be our priority. Yet so many people haven't had the opportunity to explore what happened to them, or to understand that what happened is still part of them and that these experiences are not their fault.

So as we're learning how to connect our history to our current emotional and physical health, what are some potential problem areas to keep in mind?

*Dr. Perry*: One of the most important areas is the way we connect with others. Developmental trauma can disrupt our ability to form and maintain relationships. Whenever trauma or neglect takes place in the context of our caregiving relationships, there's a high risk that the neural networks involved in reading and responding to other people will be altered. When these "attachment" capabilities are impaired, there will be difficulties with friendships, school, employment, intimacy, and family; there is even risk for repeating transgenerational patterns of abuse.

*Oprah*: It's nearly impossible for some people to go with the flow, or get along. They blow up at their boss. They're not reliable as friends. They sabotage new relationships.

*Dr. Perry*: Yet it's almost always the case that these people really do want to be connected. They may even be good at starting relationships; they're just terrible at maintaining them. And, of course, since we are, at our core, relational creatures, this difficulty is physiologically and psychologically devastating. It leads to isolation, disconnection, loneliness, and is connected to all kinds of other problems, including risk for physical health problems.

*Oprah*: Beyond the mental health community, this is why family physicians, health-care workers, and doctors in all fields need to consider not only what might be physically wrong with their patients but also what happened to them.

*Dr. Perry*: Yes. And physical health is another major potential problem area related to developmental trauma. As we've discussed, developmental adversity increases the risk for all kinds of health problems, including heart disease, asthma, gastrointestinal problems, and autoimmune disease. Understanding the correlations can change how we diagnose and treat these physical problems.

Diabetes is a great example. Worldwide there are 415 million people with the disease. In the United States, the figure is roughly 34 million—just over 1 in 10. Another 88 million American adults have prediabetic and cardiometabolic risk. If trauma has altered the CRNs (see Figure 2), there will be pervasive regulation problems, including regulation of blood sugar and insulin release. Both the risk for diabetes and the management of diabetes are related to a history of adversity.

*Oprah*: Okay, let me stop you here. Because I know there will be people who say, "Diabetes is strictly biological." But what this conversation is revealing, and what your studies for the past thirty years have proven, is that nothing is separate. Physical well-being and your emotional health are deeply connected.

*Dr. Perry*: Absolutely. I know that most people—including many doctors—make a "biological" versus "psychological" distinction when they think about health. And it is very common, for instance, for the medical community to dismiss trauma-related physical symptoms such as the headaches or abdominal pain that often afflict people with a sensitized dissociative response. Here's an example from materials on abdominal pain distributed in 2020 by an academic medical center. This is an institution that's teaching new doctors every day, and it's part of what they're still teaching: *"The vast majority of children and adolescents with recurrent* **abdominal pain** *have* **functional abdominal pain** *or 'non-organic' pain, which means the* **pain** *is not caused by physical abnormalities."*

The suggestion, of course, is that the pain is "psychosomatic" or "all in your head." This is dismissive. And indeed, many trauma-related health problems are dismissed, missed, and misunderstood. But once you understand more about neuroscience, and how our senses and brain translate experience into "biological" activity, the artificial distinctions disappear. If you understand the neurobiology of trauma, you know that a physical "abnormality" is causing the abdominal pain seen with sensitized dissociation. You begin to see that a person's "worldview" can change their immune system, and that a positive conversation with a friend can influence how a patient's heart or lungs function that day. The interconnectedness becomes clear. As you said, Oprah, *everything matters.*

Most important, you come to understand that belonging is biology, and disconnection destroys our health. Trauma is disconnecting, and that impacts every system in our body.

Let me give you an example. I was asked to do a consultation for Tyra, a hospitalized sixteen-year-old girl with diabetes. She had type 1, insulin-dependent diabetes mellitus (IDDM), sometimes called juvenile diabetes. To be clear, this form of diabetes involves both a genetic component and some exacerbating early-life experiences (for instance, infection or an autoimmune reaction). I'm not suggesting that Tyra's IDDM was caused by trauma; it was diagnosed when she was much younger, and prior to her hospitalization she had been in good control. She knew how to test her own blood sugar and give herself insulin shots.

Tyra was admitted to the hospital in a diabetic coma; her blood sugar had risen so high, she was unconscious. Her medical team addressed the crisis, and she stabilized. The next few days in the hospital were spent trying to figure out the correct insulin dose—but the medical team couldn't get it right. A dose that seemed to work in the morning turned out to be either too high (making Tyra's blood sugar crash) or too low (keeping her blood sugar dangerously high). The team began to think Tyra was intentionally manipulating her insulin or secretly eating sweets. They couldn't understand the wild swings in her blood sugar in the face of what they felt were appropriate doses of insulin. Because they suspected "self-destructive" behavior, they asked for a psychiatric consultation.

I met Tyra in her hospital room. She was positive, pleasant, cooperative, and puzzled by the medical team's inability to figure out her insulin. She had been managing her dosing well for years.

About ten minutes into our conversation, Tyra suddenly stopped talking and visibly tensed. I thought I'd done something to upset her. Then I realized she was looking out the window, in the direction of a siren from an ambulance coming to the hospital's Emergency Room. Now, if you work in a hospital setting, you hear sirens all the time, and you tune them out. I hadn't even noticed it. But Tyra had.

"May I take your heart rate?" I asked.

The question broke her stare. "Sure."

I approached, took her wrist into my hands, and took her pulse: 128 beats per minute. Very high for a young adult at rest.

"I can't help but notice that the siren seemed to be upsetting to you."

"Oh. I guess. Makes me wonder who might be hurt."

"Do you know anyone who ended up in an ambulance? Besides you, of course." The question returned her to a semi-frozen stare. I let the seconds tick by.

Eventually she blinked and started to quietly speak. "About two weeks ago, I was with some of my friends just hanging out in the park. We were sitting on a picnic table. We weren't doing anything." She stopped.

"You don't have to talk about it."

"No. It's okay." I wasn't so sure, but I let her continue.

"I didn't even really hear any gunshots. Keisha says she did. I was sitting right next to Nina, and all of a sudden she looked right at me. Her eyes got big, like this—" Tyra opened her eyes wide to show me.

"She looked all surprised—made a little squeak sound and fell over. There was blood all over her back." I could see Tyra revisiting the moment; her fear and confusion were obvious.

As the siren outside the hospital faded to nothing, she started talking again. "There were sirens and police. Took forever for the ambulance to come. They took her away. It was the middle of the day. We were just sitting there."

I took her wrist again. Her heart rate was 160 bpm. She was breathing rapidly, clearly in a state of fear (see Figure 6).

"Do your doctors know this happened?"

"I don't think so. Why would they?"

"Yeah. I guess you're right, I wouldn't expect them to ask about those things. So, Tyra, let me tell you what I think is going on with your insulin." I drew the upside-down triangle and talked about the stress response, how the body prepares to flee or fight when we feel fear.

Tyra knew a lot about how insulin helps take sugar from the blood into cells of the body, but she wasn't as aware of how adrenaline, released during distress and threat, actually "mobilizes" stored sugar reserves to assist in fight-or-flight behaviors. Adrenaline increases the sugar in your blood. Her stress response, overactivated by the recent trauma, increased her adrenaline—hence much more sugar in her blood. The dose of insulin that had worked in the past was no longer adequate. Furthermore, when she was exposed to any evocative cue, such as the sirens, her sensitized system had an overreaction, releasing very high levels of adrenaline and, in turn, leading to a huge release of sugar. So there she was, spending her days in a room where the episodic sound of sirens caused episodic blood-sugar spikes. She wasn't manipulating the insulin or sneaking food. Asking what *happened* to her changed the dynamic regulation of her blood sugar.

We moved Tyra to the other side of the hospital, where she wouldn't hear sirens at all hours of the day, and started therapy to help her heal. Within a few days, a stable insulin regimen was established, and she went home.

*Oprah*: Her doctors couldn't explain what was happening "biologically," so they assumed she was to blame. They hadn't considered that some trauma might be influencing her biology.

*Dr. Perry*: They hadn't even thought to ask. Twenty years ago, trauma was never really considered a factor in a person's health. Honestly, it was rarely considered a factor in someone's mental health. To this day, the role that trauma and developmental adversity play in mental and physical health remains underappreciated.

Children and adults with developmental trauma frequently experience chronic abdominal pain, headaches, chest pain, fainting, and seizure-like episodes—all very common symptoms related to a sensitized stress response. Most doctors, if they come up short with typical medical findings, will label these symptoms "functional" or "psychological." This kind of dismissive attitude only adds salt to the wounds.

*Oprah*: Over the years your work has really been trying to address this. One of the terms I hear you use when you teach about the brain and trauma is *sequential*. We've touched on this before, but can you explain again what that means and why it's important in appreciating "what happened" to us?

*Dr. Perry*: Of course. Anything sequential happens in a *sequence*, a set of steps—first *a*, then *b*, then *c*. And as we've said, the way our brain processes our experiences is sequential. All sensory input (physical sensations, smells, tastes, sights, sounds) is first processed in the lower areas of the brain; the lower brain gets first dibs. This means that before any new experience has a chance to be considered by the higher, "thinking" part of the brain, the lower brain has already interpreted and responded to it. It's matched the sensory input from the new experience against the catalog of stored memories of past experiences—*before* the smart part of your brain even has a chance to get involved.

But as we saw with Mike Roseman, the lower part of the brain can't "tell time." So sometimes its interpretation of incoming input is inaccurate. If any of the input is a match to a stored memory from past experience, the lower brain reacts as though the past experience is the one happening now. That's a problem when the past experience was a trauma. Mike's brain matched the sound of a motorcycle backfire to the terror of war. Tyra's brain matched the sound of sirens to the horror of her friend's death. For you, Oprah, being alone at night triggered the sensory memory of that night so many years ago with your grandfather's attack.

## Figure 10

## SEQUENCE OF ENGAGEMENT

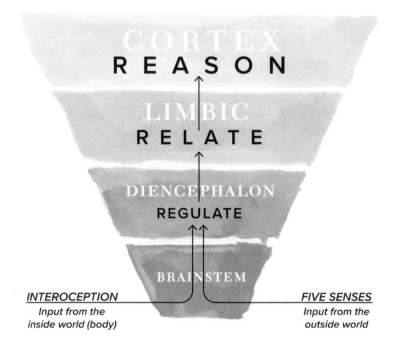

CORTEX
**R E A S O N**

LIMBIC
**R E L A T E**

DIENCEPHALON
**REGULATE**

BRAINSTEM

*INTEROCEPTION*
*Input from the
inside world (body)*

*FIVE SENSES*
*Input from the
outside world*

Our brain is continually getting input from our body (interoception) and the world (five senses). These incoming signals are processed in a sequential fashion, with the first sorting taking place in the lower brain (brainstem, diencephalon). To reason with another person, we need to effectively get through the lower areas of their brain and reach their cortex, the part responsible for thinking, including problem-solving and reflective cognition. But if someone is stressed, angry, frustrated, or otherwise dysregulated, the incoming input will be short-circuited, leading to inefficient, distorted input to the cortex. This is where the sequence of engagement comes in. Without some degree of regulation, it is difficult to connect with another person, and without connection, there is minimal reasoning. Regulate, relate, then reason. Trying to reason with someone before they are regulated won't work and indeed will only increase frustration (dysregulation) for both of you. Effective communication, teaching, coaching, parenting, and therapeutic input require awareness of, and adherence to, the sequence of engagement.

*Oprah*: So the brain interprets two experiences similarly even though they may have happened decades apart. You might see them as separate events, but your brain categorizes them as the same. You describe this as a sort of miscommunication within the brain.

*Dr. Perry*: Yes. And understanding that our brain processes every experience sequentially also helps explain miscommunication *between* brains— in other words, between people. Communication, after all, is about getting some idea, concept, or story from your cortex to another person's cortex. From the smart part of your brain to the smart part of their brain. The problem is that we don't communicate directly from cortex to cortex. We have to go through the lower parts of the brain. All the rational thoughts from our cortex have to get through the emotional filters of the lower brain. Our facial expression, tone of voice, and words are turned into neural activity by the other person's senses, and then the sequential process of matching, interpreting, and passing up to their cortex takes place. Along the way, there are many opportunities for the meaning of any communication to be distilled, distorted, magnified, minimized, or lost.

Let's think about what happens when the stress response is activated. Frustration, anger, and fear can shut down parts of the cortex. When someone is dysregulated, they simply cannot use the smartest part of their brain. Look back at Figure 6, which illustrates state-dependent functioning; the further you move along the "arousal" continuum, the more the lower parts of the brain dominate your functioning.

In my work we talk about "getting to the cortex"—getting to the place where you can communicate rationally with someone. If the person is regulated, you can connect with them in ways that will facilitate rational communication. But if they're dysregulated, nothing you say will really get to their cortex, and nothing already in their cortex will be easy for them to access. This is essential to understand if you're a teacher, because while the regulated child can learn, the dysregulated child will not. But it's the same for supervising people in a work setting or communicating with colleagues, your partner, your children—anyone. Regulation is the key to creating a safe connection. And being connected is the most efficient and effective way to get information up to the cortex. A tutor, a coach, a mentor, a therapist—all depend on the relationship to be the superhighway to the cortex.

We use the term *sequence of engagement* to describe the steps involved in getting to the cortex. Let me give you an example of a real-life application of this sequence.

Over the years I have had the opportunity to work with law enforcement, including the Federal Bureau of Investigation (FBI), mostly teaching about the effects of trauma and interviewing children. For a time, I did more active consulting for the FBI's Child Abduction and Serial Killer Task Force. In this role I was occasionally asked to interview children—victims and witnesses.

Joseph was a three-year-old child who had witnessed his eleven-year-old sister's abduction several weeks earlier. At the time of the abduction, the two of them were out playing in their neighborhood, in the middle of the afternoon. When Joseph ran home, all he could say to his mother was that "the man took Sissy." A week later her body was found.

Local law enforcement and the FBI had interviewed Joseph, but this young, overwhelmed boy was unable to give many details about "the man" or the abduction.

Interviewing three-year-old children is challenging under any circumstances, and I was a complete stranger prying into the most painful experience of Joseph's life. I knew that any useful information was going to be stored in "narrative" memory—essentially, his mental reconstruction of the event. Key elements of narrative memory are stored in higher parts of the brain, especially the cortex.

I also knew that fear inhibits many cortical systems, in effect shutting them down; this includes those involved in narrative memory (see Figure 11). Joseph would never be able to give me any useful information if he didn't feel safe.

Aware of the power of social contagion (remember flocking?), I reasoned that if Joseph's mother could send signals of acceptance and familiarity when I was around, he would feel safer with me; this is the brain's version of "any friend of yours is a friend of mine."

Another thing that contributes to feeling safe with another person is a history of positive experiences with that person. The more positive time you spend with someone, the more your brain categorizes that person as safe and familiar. This is why, in therapy, it often takes ten to twenty sessions before the client begins to feel safe enough to share some of their most emotionally difficult experiences. With a "dose" of fifty minutes once a week, the traditional therapeutic process would take ten weeks for Joseph to feel safe with me. That wasn't practical for this kind of interview.

So how to become—quickly—safe and familiar to Joseph? How to make the networks in his brain categorize me as safe? As we discussed with the little boy who'd witnessed his mother's death in a home invasion, a meaningful "dose"—or period of activation—for neural networks is only seconds long. So rather than have ten fifty-minute therapy sessions to allow Joseph to make a set of memories about me, I would have ten or twelve five-minute interactions. Engage, connect, clarify, disengage: five minutes. Engage, connect, play, disengage: five minutes. Go in and out of his visual field, his space, keeping in mind all the factors that can impact anyone's feeling of safety in any interaction. My brief interactions had to minimize any dysregulating elements and maximize regulating and connecting elements.

Part of the problem here was the natural "power differential" that exists between an adult and a child. In every person-to-person interaction there are complex calculations going on in each person's brain: *Is this person safe? Are they an ally or enemy? Will they hurt me or help me? What are they planning to do? What are they trying to do? What do they want?* This relational calculus helps define where we are in a power differential. *We are equal: I don't feel threatened. I am dominant:*

# Figure 11

## STATE DEPENDENCE AND MEMORY

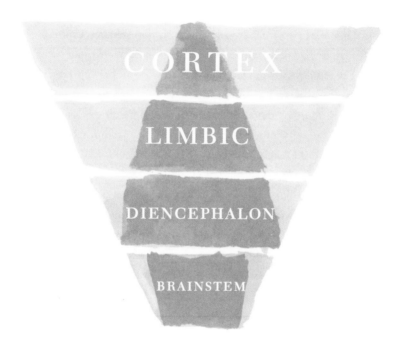

**DYSREGULATED** ————————

**Inefficient access to
cortical memories**

---

### STATE DEPENDENCE AND ACCESS TO 'NARRATIVE' MEMORY

In a fear state (dysregulated), there is a "shutdown" of some of the systems in higher areas of the brain (e.g., cortical). This makes retrieval of previous linear narrative memory inefficient; a common example of this is test anxiety. The content has been stored, but in the moment (e.g., during the test), retrieval is not possible. When the person is regulated, and feeling connected and safe, the stored content is accessible and easier to retrieve.

CORTEX

LIMBIC

DIENCEPHALON

BRAINSTEM

1. Regulate
2. Relate
3. Reason

→ **REGULATED**

**Cortical memories
accessible**

*I am safe. They are dominant: I am vulnerable.* If we feel vulnerable, there will be a state-dependent shift in our stress-response systems—and therefore in how we feel, think, and interpret the interaction.

This relational calculus is for keeping us safe and alive. If we don't feel safe, we become dysregulated. The implications of this are profound, by the way; these dynamics of power are built into our sociopolitical systems and play a key role in, for example, systemic racism.

*Oprah*: I remember you explaining the power differential in terms of the person whose voice is interpreted differently. For me specifically, while we were talking about leadership challenges at OWLAG, you said, "Your whisper is heard as a shout." That was an *Aha*.

*Dr. Perry*: Well, you *are* the Oprah effect. When you're on the top of a power differential, sometimes you don't realize the power you have—or the impact your mere presence can have on others. We'll talk about this a lot when we talk about healing.

In this case, imagine a six-foot-two man talking to a three-foot child about a man murdering his sister—the power differential was going to be huge. If I was going to "get to his cortex," I had to work to decrease that differential.

After talking with the FBI agents, the mother, and members of my team, we set up the interview to take place in Joseph's home, where he felt safest. As we started, the mother and I sat at the kitchen table talking while Joseph warily wandered in and out of the room. The mother had been asked to introduce me.

"Joseph, come here, honey," she said. "Meet my friend, Dr. Perry."

With trepidation, Joseph approached. I got off my chair and got down on the floor with him. I was trying to minimize the obvious physical difference, make myself smaller, and get eye-to-eye.

"Hi, Joseph. I'm Dr. Perry. I came to visit your mom and you." He looked at me. Because the unknown fuels fear, I wanted him to know who, what, why. "I'm a doctor who works with children who have had hard things happen to their family. Your mom told me about your sister. I'm so sorry." Joseph stopped moving and stared into space. "Today you and I are going to play. And later, when you are ready, I will ask a few questions about your sister." Then I stood up.

"I'm going to go get some coffee," I said. "Do you want anything?" Joseph didn't look at me and didn't say a word.

I asked his mother. "Sure," she said. "I'll have some coffee."

All of this had taken about three minutes. I walked out the front door. Ten minutes later, I was back. I sat and talked with the mother for another ten minutes, while Joseph again wandered in and out of the kitchen, now getting closer to the kitchen table each time. There were a few toy trucks on the living room floor. I got down on the floor and started to play with one. Initially, Joseph ignored me, but then came over and cautiously pulled the truck away from me.

"I'm sorry, Joseph. I should have asked to use your truck." He sat a few feet away and pretended to play with the truck. Then I got up, said, "I have to go run an errand, but I'll be back"—and left again.

After about ten minutes, I came back, this time with crayons and paper. I sat at the kitchen table silently coloring. Joseph's mother sat with me, sipping her coffee. Curious, Joseph came over and watched. I didn't look at him but slowly held my hand out with a crayon and a piece of paper. He didn't take it.

I got down on the living room floor and took the crayons and paper. Joseph brought the truck over and held it out. I took it and gave him some paper and a crayon. He lay on his stomach next to me, and we colored silently for about five minutes. Then I got up, and he looked directly at me, as if to question where I was going. "I will be back. Can you take care of these colors for me?"

"Yes." His first word.

This went on for about three more brief sessions. At one point, Joseph said, "Here are my best toys." He took my hand and walked me into his bedroom. We went through his whole collection. He was talking in full sentences, conversational, comfortable. I'd been able to get him regulated, through play, patterned repetitive coloring, relational endorsement from Mom, walking, and talking. And with the back-and-forth engagements, his brain's facial recognition systems categorized me as familiar. There had been a dozen "episodes" of interaction; those systems didn't really register that these were all part of the same four-hour visit.

Joseph and I were connected; I was perceived as safe and familiar. His cortical networks and narrative memory were accessible. Could he talk about his sister's abduction without shutting down?

I gave him control. "Remember what I said about talking about your sister?"

"Yes." Joseph nodded and stopped playing.

"We don't have to talk about this if you don't want to."

"Okay," Joseph said, but didn't resume playing.

I asked if he remembered what the man looked like. He gave a few details. I needed more—long hair, short hair, mustache, clothes, thin, heavy? I took an old newspaper to use pictures of men as examples, unaware that the paper contained photos related to his sister's abduction.

He saw a picture of her. "That's Sissy. She's dead."

I pointed to different advertisements—"Did he have hair like this?"—attempting to get more detail. Then I turned the page, and Joseph's posture changed.

Looking at a picture of a suspect, he sat forward. "That's him," he said. "That's the bad guy. He has glasses."

When shown multiple photos of other men with similar features, Joseph all but ignored them. Later, he immediately identified the suspect from a virtual lineup of men all having similar features.

At the end of the interview, I said, "Joseph, do you remember where the man took your sister?"

"Yes."

"Can you take me there?"

As we walked through his neighborhood, Joseph narrated what had happened. His sister had been bouncing his ball; it had fallen into a deep ditch on the side of the road. As he went to get it, a red truck drove up, a man got out, took his sister into the cab. The man never saw Joseph.

As he relived the experience, Joseph became visibly upset. He'd had enough. We stopped, but his identification and description of the abduction led directly to evidence instrumental in the conviction of his sister's murderer.

*Oprah*: You got to his cortex.

*Dr. Perry*: Yes. Joseph's story is a good example of the sequence of engagement. In order to communicate rationally and successfully with anyone, you have to make sure they're *regulated,* make sure they feel a *relationship* with you, and only then try to *reason* with them. Twenty years ago, I knew enough about this—and about the impact of stress and trauma on the brain in general—to be able to communicate with Joseph without causing his cortex to shut down. But when I walked out of his house, I left a broken family. The pain of the traumatic loss of a daughter remained for the mother; for Joseph, a big sister would always be gone. Every year there is a hollow birthday for Sissy; empty places at the family table every holiday; Mother's Day is painful and bittersweet.

We didn't yet know enough about healing. Though we worked with hundreds of families, and though I could have given a pretty good explanation of what I thought was causing their pain, exhaustion, depression, anxiety, intrusive images, even their dysregulated health—I just didn't really know how to make any of it much better. But we kept listening and learning.

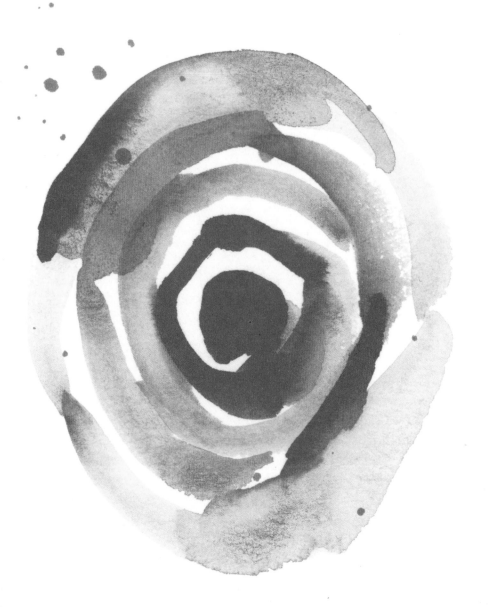

# CHAPTER 6

# FROM COPING TO HEALING

*I've spent most of my career trying to understand how stress and trauma change us. But when I was just getting started, I was overfocused on extreme traumatic events. Hundreds and ultimately thousands of children, youth, and adults shared their life stories with me. I listened and reflected on how what I was hearing fit with the extensive neuroscience research on stress in animals. Many times I thought,* Ah, now I understand. This is how trauma works. This is how trauma influences the brain and behavior. *But I was wrong. I was learning important things, but I didn't understand, not completely.*

*I started to think more deeply about healing after trauma. I had believed that if a person's trauma history was more extreme, healing would be more difficult. But there were pieces of the puzzle I wasn't seeing.*

*This became apparent to me thirty years ago, when I was trying to understand two boys, both twelve years old, living at a residential treatment center. Each had been sent there because they'd been "out of control" in a series of foster homes and other residential schools. They were both in the sixth grade, but both struggled in school, reading at a fourth-grade level. When I reviewed their records, both had the same DSM labels: ADHD, major depression, intermittent explosive disorder, and conduct disorder. They were both on multiple medications, prescribed as attempts to curb their disruptive symptoms. And both had been in the residential program for about a year.*

*But when I met them, I "felt" different sitting with each one. Both created a mood in the room, but each created a completely different emotional climate. Thomas had suffered physical abuse at the hands of an explosive, rageful father. At age six he was removed from his home. He had been through twelve foster homes, and three hospitalizations eventually led to placement at this residential center. The year he'd been at the center was the longest he'd ever lived anywhere in his life. He continued to have visits with his mother and occasionally with his father. Despite his history, he was interactive, he smiled,* and he tried to help me get to know him. But his hypervigilance, restlessness, and extreme mood swings were easy to see. When we first met, his resting HR was 128 bpm. His inattentive, oppositional, defiant, and aggressive behaviors were manifestations of an overactive and overly reactive arousal response (see Figures 5 and 6). He was in a persistent state of fear. I didn't believe it was useful to think of his having four separate DSM disorders; he had one—a childhood version of PTSD.

James had a completely different "feel"—actually, it was no feel at all. It was as if I were sitting with a ghost, as if he were empty. When I was with him, I felt alone. His records indicated none of the more "traditional" traumatic events common in foster children. His mother, likely struggling with depression, had disappeared with a boyfriend when James was three months old. After he'd spent six weeks in "shelter care," his maternal grandmother, who lived alone, agreed to take him. It seems that she was not happy about having to raise James. The picture that emerged from reviewing the old records was of a demoralized and bitter caregiver. But she did her best. There was no history of physical abuse, sexual abuse, exposure to drug-using behavior, or other forms of trauma; multiple records simply documented a disengaged, "exhausted," non-interactive style of child rearing, and minimal verbal or physical interactions. In his grandmother's care, James started to be inattentive and disobedient. Rewards didn't seem to work, and consequences didn't seem to bother him. He would take seemingly meaningless things from others—a pencil, a bracelet, a small toy. When confronted about these thefts, he would deny them, even in the face of clear evidence. Several times he'd threatened to stab other students, and he was described as having explosive aggression, but on closer examination, he never actually hit, pushed, or attacked anyone. He only threatened.

At age eight, James's grandmother ran out of gas and simply quit. She abandoned him "to the system" because he was "lying, stealing, ungrateful," and she was becoming afraid of him. James had threatened to kill her in her sleep. He entered the child protection system and bounced from foster home to foster home before ending up at this residential setting. The inattentiveness that led to his ADHD diagnosis wasn't the vigilant, distractible kind like Thomas's. James was inattentive because he was disengaged and daydreaming. In contrast to Thomas's resting HR of 128, James's was 60 bpm.

Despite being given the same DSM labels, Thomas and James were nothing alike. I started to wonder about James as an infant. A young, inexperienced mother, struggling with depression, overwhelmed by the nonstop needs of a baby. Maybe his mother had some relational or attachment issues—what had happened to her? You can't give what you don't have.

Imagine an early childhood in which James's mom meets his needs, but maybe not much more. Just as he is beginning to organize his "relational" neurobiology, his whole world changes, and a new set of adults starts caring for him at the shelter. Each of these adults has a different smell, voice, style of touch. And then suddenly they are all gone, too. James, five months old, with a rapidly developing brain containing a set of confused, disorganized "memories" about human connection, has learned that people disappear. They are not consistent or predictable. They do not reliably meet his needs, comfort him, reward him.

Now imagine any hungry, scared, cold infant and an episodically responsive caregiver. The infant's version of the fight-or-flight response is to cry. But if crying doesn't bring the responsive caregiver, or if the crying brings a frustrated or enraged caregiver, the infant is forced to use other self-soothing options. An infant's dominant adaptive response to stress in these situations is to disengage from the confusing, threatening outside world and retreat into their inner world.

When I met James, I knew that dissociation was the primary adaptation when animals were stressed in specific ways—when the threat was inescapable or immobilizing and when fighting was useless. This kind of stress leads to a "capitulation" or "defeat" response in animals. Their physiology changes. They play dead. The animal research in this area is extensive. Oddly, to this day, parallel research into the neurophysiology of dissociation in humans lags well behind.

In any case, here were two children with the same DSM labels, but with different behaviors and different responses to treatment. Where did the differences come from? From what happened to them as children.

As I spent more time with Thomas, I started to hear more about all the loving people in his tumultuous world. His mother, aunt, and maternal grandmother were all very affectionate and continued to try to get the system to let Thomas come home. But his mother would not leave her husband. And the husband couldn't stop using.

I learned that Thomas's father had not always been abusive. His struggles, according to the family, started after he came back from Vietnam. Back then, PTSD was not well understood, and many Vietnam vets received no help at all. The father's alcohol and drug use led to his getting fired; as he became unable to care for his family, his self-esteem collapsed. The trauma cycle—shame, pain, booze, rage, humiliation, and loss—accelerated the family's fragmentation.

Before his father's deterioration, Thomas had had a good start in life, with loving and consistent caregiving. When he was an infant, his father wasn't abusive. But as his father struggled, his family suffered, especially his mom. Thomas's father started to beat him when Thomas tried to protect his mother. And then he became the major lightning rod for his father's rage. But while his mother and other family members were unable to protect him completely, they did what they could. The buffering effect of these caregivers and his good early start made all the difference. Thomas ended up with healthy relational neurobiology despite his trauma-sensitized stress response.

*Thomas improved with treatment. His healthy relational capabilities allowed him to do very well with a relationally focused therapeutic process. Within twelve months, he was much less dysregulated. He was able to focus and learn more easily. He had far fewer behavioral problems and advanced two grade levels in one year. He started to heal.*

*James did not improve at the same pace. In fact, he got worse. His predatory behaviors continued, and he grew smarter at not getting caught. All efforts to shape his behavior or build healthy relationships failed. It was almost as if, even with therapeutic help, he didn't have the tools to succeed.*

*As we will talk about much more, relationships are the key to healing. But for James, every relational interaction resulted in disengagement. To him, "others" were not safe. In his worldview, people hurt you or left you. Others could not be trusted. The lesson for me was that a key aspect of* What happened to you? *is* What didn't *happen for you? What attention, nurturing touch, reassurance—basically, what love— didn't you get? I realized that neglect is as toxic as trauma.*

—Dr. Perry

*Oprah*: When you say *neglect,* what do you mean? Isn't neglect traumatic?

*Dr. Perry*: I do think that, in most cases, neglect and trauma co-occur. But they cause very different biological experiences and can have very different effects on the brain and the developing child. Some people have used the term "complex trauma" to try to capture developmental neglect and maltreatment, but I believe that lumps too many things into one box.

*Oprah*: So help me understand neglect.

*Dr. Perry*: Okay, let's think about the developing child. In order for the genetic potential of that child to be expressed, a variety of necessary experiences is required.

If these experiences are absent, or if their timing, pattern, or nature is abnormal, key capabilities do not develop. Neglect is most destructive early in life, when the brain is rapidly growing; early neglect interferes with the child's getting the necessary stimulation required for normal development.

You've probably heard of the "Romanian orphans." It is likely that more than five hundred thousand children spent part of their early lives in the state-run institutional orphanages during the Ceaușescu regime in Romania; in 1989, when communism ended in the country, the public and press saw the horrible conditions these children had been subjected to. There were often forty to sixty babies or toddlers in a single large room, each in their own crib all day long, with only one or two caregivers rotating among them over the course of a twelve-hour shift. The children suffered deprivation, malnutrition, abuse, and more. Even after being removed from the institutions, they grew up with a range of deficits. Some had low IQs, others couldn't walk, most had major problems forming and maintaining relationships. I worked with many children removed from these orphanages. In general, the longer the child was there, the longer the deprivation, the more serious the problems. Ironically, in some overcrowded institutions, children who had to share cribs ultimately did better.

The Romanian orphans are now adults; for most of them, problems persist. As a group they are much more likely to be unemployed, have mental and physical health problems, and have difficulties with relationships.

Similar isolated cases have happened in the United States, and our clinical group has worked with many children and youth who've emerged from extremely neglectful backgrounds. These children grow up undersocialized. They have no toilet training, cannot use utensils, have minimal language skills. In the most extreme cases, they appear "wild"; the term used is *feral*.

You actually highlighted the story of one of these children, Dani, the "girl in the window," on *The Oprah Winfrey Show*. She was locked up and profoundly neglected for the first six years of her life, with tragic results. Fortunately, she was removed and adopted. Her healing journey has been agonizingly slow, but steady.

*Oprah*: When she got into a loving home, she started to get better. But she continued to struggle with communication and social interactions.

*Dr. Perry*: She struggles to this day. So many important things happen in the developing brain of a child in the first six years of life. And if key neural networks do not get the right "experiences" at the right times, some essential capabilities will not develop normally. We still have so much to learn about this, and we know that other developmental factors, such as intrauterine insults or birth trauma, may be involved in extreme cases like Dani's. But as seen with the Romanian orphans, the longer you spend in a deprived developmental environment, the harder it will be to recover.

*Oprah*: But these examples, like Dani, are so uncommon. Six years is such a long time. What happens if it's only one year? What if it's only when one specific babysitter comes over? What if you ground a teenager and they basically have to stay in their room for a month? Is that neglect?

*Dr. Perry*: Grounding a teenager is not neglect, because key systems in the brain have already developed. I'm not advocating that you send a fifteen-year-old to their room for a month, but it isn't the same as a month of deprivation in early childhood.

But the issues you raise are important ones. And just as with trauma, several essential questions can help us assess whether a situation is neglectful, and if so, how great its impact will be. When during development did the neglect take place? What was the pattern? How severe or depriving was the neglect? How long did it last? And, since absolute total neglect is rare, what "buffering" factors were present when the neglect occurred?

The most common form of neglect is fragmented, patternless caregiving. Some days when the infant cries, adults come to feed and nurture them. Other days, no one comes. Still other days, someone comes and yells at, shakes, or hurts them. This confusing, chaotic world is very dysregulating. The infant gets insufficient "structure" to send a clear, organized set of signals to the developing systems in the brain. The infant's world is unpredictable, and the result is a "chaotic" neglect. Key systems develop in a fragmented, disorganized way, leading to functional problems.

Another kind of neglect—"splinter" neglect—occurs when many aspects of development are normal and some key systems receive appropriately timed experiences, but one or more does not—leading to the absence of a critical aspect of healthy development. Let me give you an example.

I once worked with five siblings, ages eleven, eight, six, four, and two. They were all delightful. Their mother was raising them on her own; she had two doctoral degrees and loved her children very much. The problem was that she had a fixed delusion and a profound fear that her children would be harmed if they left her sight. So she started to keep the children in the same room with her—all the children, all day, all night. Over time she started to home-school, and she insisted that the children sit in car seats on the couches. She got to the point where she kept them in physical restraint in the car seats. Didn't let them crawl or walk.

She was warm to these children, and very focused on their cognitive development. All the children were two or more academic grades advanced. They were verbal and socially interactive with one another, but even the oldest child could barely stand up. There had been a "splinter" deprivation of motor activity; the result was a family of children with grossly underdeveloped legs and neuromotor capabilities. This is an extreme example of splinter neglect. But there are many other examples where one important domain of development is relatively ignored or understimulated, including emotional development.

*Oprah*: There are different ways to neglect a child. I've seen children grow up neglected because they were unseen in the household. Emotional ghosts, like James.

*Dr. Perry*: Oh, yes. I've worked with several emotionally neglected children of very wealthy parents who chose to "outsource" parenting but did so in a way that was developmentally uninformed. They didn't understand the importance of relational consistency early in life, so their infant was cared for by different shifts of hired caregivers.

*Oprah*: What do you mean by that? There is a lot of messaging in the world that tells us it doesn't matter who or how many people are caring for a child as long as that child is receiving love and attention. Is that wrong?

*Dr. Perry*: That's a great question. In general, the more attentive and loving people in your life, the better. But if you remember our earlier discussions about the developing brain and the process of creating your worldview, you'll remember that early in life, the brain needs consistent, patterned experiences to develop some key systems. Let's look at language development to illustrate what I mean.

Say you speak only English to an infant for six weeks and then say, "English is done, we're going to speak Chinese." For the next five months, the child hears only Chinese, but then, "We're done with Chinese, now we're going to speak French." And the language spoken to the child changes ten more times before they turn three. This poor child will not speak any language at all. Despite the fact that these are good languages, and that all the languages "activate" the speech and language part of the brain, there were never sufficient repetitions with any one language to properly organize the child's full speech and language capability.

Language disruptions would also take place if the child heard fifteen different languages spoken each day. There would be insufficient time and insufficient repetitions with any one language for the infant's developing brain to make sense of any of the languages. Language development would be delayed and possibly abnormal.

It's the same thing with relationships. If you familiarize with one person for six weeks and then they disappear and a new person starts caring for you, and then that person disappears, and so on, your infant brain hasn't had sufficient repetitions with any single person to create the architecture that allows you to develop healthy relational neurobiology.

The key to having many healthy relationships in your life is having only a few safe, stable, and nurturing relationships in your first year. This lets you get adequate repetitions to build the foundation—the fundamental relational architecture—that will allow you to continue to grow healthy relational connections. Again, think of language:

Once you've learned one or two primary languages, you can go on to learn many others. But when an infant, toddler, or child grows up in a household where "loving" is outsourced, the result can be a form of splinter neglect, where key relational capabilities are undeveloped or stunted.

*Oprah*: And I think as we become more and more dependent on technology in so many aspects of our lives, one big aspect is the care of our children. More and more, I see parents outsourcing childcare to the phone or tablet. Or the children are left to their own metaphorical devices while the parents are distracted by their literal devices. Once when I was driving in Chicago, my car ended up behind a horse-drawn carriage. The children were leaning out and looking around. The mother was on her phone chitty-chatting away. For the entire ride. Not once did she engage with the children or even look at them. And I kept thinking, *When they're done, she'll post a picture saying, Look at us, wasn't that great, we did the horse and carriage ride.* I see this so often now: parents who are with their children but not really *with* them.

*Dr. Perry*: I think this is a huge problem in our distracted society. We are not very good at truly being present.

*Oprah*: And even a baby can tell when you're there. They know if you are excited or happy. They can feel it. They know if they are safe or not. They want eye contact.

*Dr. Perry*: They want full engagement. They want you to be present. The inability to be really present has a toxic impact on healthy development. As we've talked about earlier, the infant's brain is trying to make sense of the world, and because we are social creatures, a crucial part of this is building a sense of belonging: *I matter, I'm one of the clan.* This comes from getting specific "you matter" signals from others, especially your family. And it requires giving the infant, toddler, or child your attention. Not partial attention—fully engaged attention. *I'm looking at you. I'm listening. I'm right here with you.*

All of us have had the experience of having a conversation with somebody and feeling dismissed when they disengage to look at their phone. And even though we're adults and we have developed brains and we understand how the world works, it still feels disrespectful. It hurts.

*Oprah*: It feels like, *I wasn't important enough to hold your attention.*

*Dr. Perry*: Exactly. *I am not important enough.* It's bad enough to get that message from someone when you are an adult, just imagine if this is a constant message the baby gets when they are creating their "worldview": *I'm not important.* The infant's capability to be empathic and nurturing—their capacity to love—depends upon the nature, quality, and number of loving interactions they experience early in life. A dismissive, disengaged interaction is not building the foundation for a loving person. On the contrary, it's building the foundation for an emotionally hungry, needy person who will long for belonging but won't have the neurobiological capability to really find what they need. Dismissive caregiving can lead to an unquenchable thirst for love. You cannot love if you have not been loved.

*Oprah*: From a scientific perspective, what is happening when a mom or dad is on their cell phone while the child is attempting to have a shared experience with them?

*Dr. Perry*: There's a famous experiment in developmental psychology created by a friend and colleague of mine, Dr. Ed Tronick, called the Still-Face paradigm, which can give us a clue. In brief, a parent is instructed to not give any expression when interacting with their baby. They are asked to be disengaged, passive, and cool toward the child. The infant immediately tries to engage the parent and, within seconds of being unsuccessful, becomes significantly distressed.

*Oprah*: They start crying?

*Dr. Perry*: Often they do. The Still-Face paradigm shows viscerally that within seconds of a child perceiving their parent to be disengaged and emotionally absent, they start to feel distress and attempt to reengage the parent. But when these efforts fail, the infant disengages and emotionally withdraws. Imagine the impact on a developing child if that is a continuous experience. A cold, disengaged, partially attentive caregiver can have immediate, and potentially lifelong, toxic effects on the developing child. This child may grow up feeling inadequate, unlovable. Even with many gifts and skills, they will feel they are "not enough" as an adult, and that can lead to a host of maladaptive behaviors including unhealthy forms of attention seeking, self-sabotaging, or even self-destructive behavior.

*Oprah*: And when a young child depends on their parent or caregiver to regulate them, and that caregiver is dismissive, disengaged, or even absent when the infant needs comfort or food, this is creating that pattern of stress activation for the infant that is unpredictable and uncontrollable.

*Dr. Perry*: Yes, and that creates a sensitized stress response (see Figure 3). Let's talk about that; we know the human body—whether you are an infant or an adult—has several systems that help you deal with whatever challenge you're facing in the moment. The one most people are familiar with is the fight-or-flight response, which we've talked about (see Figure 6).

*Oprah*: So I'm looking at this figure—calm, alert, alarm, fear, terror. Walk me through this.

*Dr. Perry*: When we are stressed there is a graded response, gradually activating the systems in the brain and body that will help us. When you are not under any stress, you can be *Calm;* you can reflect on the past, the future. But as soon as you have any challenge— say a presentation at work—you enter a state of *Alert.* You scan the crowd, study faces as you present, trying to gauge if your point is being made. *Do they get this? Do they like my presentation? Are they bored?* And later in the day, you get into a small fender bender, and for a moment you enter the *Alarm* state; you're kind of frozen, not sure what to do. . . . *Should I call my insurance? Do I need to report this to the police? Should I get his information?* You're temporarily in brain freeze—when suddenly, the other driver jumps out of his car and starts screaming and threatening you with a gun. Now you enter a state of full-blown *Fear.*

And this is also where another major component of your stress-response capabilities kicks in: dissociation. Your brain is continually monitoring the situation and constantly assessing options: *Am I going to be able to run away from this? Am I going to be able to win this fight?* Your brain says you can't win a fight with a guy who's got a gun, so you start to try avoiding additional conflict, and apologize profusely. You have a sensation of watching this happen to you as if you are in a movie. You are so robotically compliant with his demands that you pay him on the spot. Your sense of time distorts. You are dissociating. Your body is preparing for potential injury; your heart rate drops. Instead of all of your blood going to your muscles to help fight or flee, you constrict peripheral blood flow. You can get pale or even faint. Your body is preparing you for injury by disconnecting you from the threat of the outside world, and bringing you into your inner world. Your body releases endogenous opioids—endorphins, enkephalin—your own natural painkiller, and you literally have the sensation that you are watching something happen to you.

*Oprah:* And that's what people describe as an "out-of-body experience" and very often don't fully remember what happens next.

*Dr. Perry:* Precisely. This dissociative response is used when there is inescapable, unavoidable distress and pain. Your mind and body protect you. Because you cannot physically flee, and fighting is futile, you psychologically flee to your inner world. So going back to the infant with a disengaged parent; the infant's fight-or-flight response is to cry. But if no one comes—or they come and are angry—the helpless infant will dissociate to survive this inescapable distressing situation. The same is true for children, youth, and adults faced with any inescapable, unavoidable pain and distress; they dissociate. And a whole set of neurophysiological changes helps you do that, including the release of your body's own opiates.

*Oprah:* Is that why people say, "Everything slowed down"?

*Dr. Perry:* That's right. When you are in that dissociative state, your sense of time dissolves. Experiences that are only seconds long can seem like minutes. Minutes can feel like you are trapped in a timeless moment.

I have debriefed FBI agents after shootings, for example. An agent might take eight minutes to describe an event that was actually ten seconds long. And it's because in that moment their brain is floating. They're out of their body watching something happen.

Many of us can connect with that feeling if we have ever experienced grief, which can elicit a feeling of numbness. We sometimes robotically go through the motions of daily living or have moments where we feel as if we are in a movie.

*Oprah*: I'm fascinated by what you're saying because I've often wondered, for example, about the people who were on the airplanes on 9/11. They knew there was a terrorist and that they only had moments to call their families. In that moment of terror, there must have been some sense of dissociation because many were able to still function enough to call family, or write a note, or rush the cockpit.

*Dr. Perry*: What you are pointing out is how adaptive it is to partially dissociate in many situations. If a soldier in combat simply went down the arousal continuum—and got to the flee and then fight stages—he would jump up and get shot. In order to maintain access to parts of his cortex—to think and behave in the ways he was trained to keep him alive in combat—he needs to dissociate to a certain degree. It's critical to survival. Without dissociation, the more a person is threatened, the more fearful they become, and the more the cortex shuts down. Being able to partially dissociate, to disengage from parts of the external threatening world and focus on trained behaviors, is key to success in competitive sport or high-pressure performances in the arts. The terms "flow" and "in the zone" are used to describe some of these partial dissociative states.

*Oprah*: In reality, everyone uses dissociation every day. That's what daydreaming is, right? And it can be a healthy coping mechanism.

*Dr. Perry*: Exactly—mind-wandering. Reflective thinking and creativity require that we stop in the middle of a moment, reflect, and spend time "in our head." We reflect on the past and imagine the future, making dissociative disengagement a key part of daily life. And it's essential for relational interaction, as well.

*Oprah*: I was surprised when you told me that most people can only be completely focused on someone and what they are saying for about fifteen seconds, and then the mind wanders. It focuses in and out on how what the other person is saying relates to something else in the listener's life, and how that connects to something else, and back and forth.

*Dr. Perry*: And that's a very normal and adaptive capability. We should understand that dissociation is not a bad thing, though it can happen in bad circumstances. Dissociating itself is a good thing. For example, a child daydreaming in class can indicate creativity. Our current public education system is good at producing workers, but it can be a miserable place for creators, artists, and future leaders.

*Oprah*: Very often we punish the child who's daydreaming.

*Dr. Perry*: We do. But in a developmentally informed, trauma-aware school, there is an understanding that downtime plays a crucial role for memory consolidation. Dissociative reflection is encouraged.

*Oprah*: Ah, yes. I'm very much aware of this principle of dissociation because of my school in South Africa. The girls there are brilliant— you've met many of them. But they come from challenged, trauma-tized backgrounds, and we had to train our teachers to understand that daydreaming or dissociation is actually good for them. It's an expected coping mechanism when you're raised in an environment where there's inescapable chaos and minimal support or other ways to keep yourself regulated. You need to be able to shut yourself down. You need to dissociate from that environment and its intensity in order to survive.

*Dr. Perry*: Exactly. Dissociation as a coping mechanism will happen more commonly when the individual feels that a threatening situation is inescapable. If you're a child and your family has a lot of conflict, you don't have many options. You can't say, "Hey, I'm moving out." Very young children can't fight or flee. They have to stay.

*Oprah*: At what point does dissociation as a coping mechanism become dissociative disorder, where the child increasingly takes herself to her inner world?

*Dr. Perry*: You kind of nailed it earlier when you talked about the infant with the disengaged parent. Remember that a pattern of stress that is unpredictable, uncontrollable, and prolonged will sensitize the stress-response systems. And if dissociation is your preferred mode of stress adaptation for long periods of time when you're young, you end up with a sensitized dissociative response to any challenge. The dissociative response is overactive and overly reactive.

Some of the young women at OWLAG, for example, after growing up in chaos and threat as young girls, would dissociate in the face of any challenge. When faced with any discomfort whatsoever.

*Oprah*: I think this part of our discussion is going to be helpful to a lot of people who wonder why they tend to check out. *Why can't I stay in the game when things get challenging?* It's because your brain has been trained to dissociate when things become uncomfortable or feel like a threat to you. Even if a math test isn't as big a threat as someone who wants to harm you, your dissociative response may be so overly reactive that your response to the math test is to shut down.

*Dr. Perry*: Right. But the response is not always a complete shutdown. As we have discussed before, the dissociative response to challenges and threats happens on a continuum (see Figure 6). For individuals who tend to have a dissociative response to stress, the first stage in the continuum is avoidance. These people don't want conflict. They want to be invisible. Avoid eye contact. Don't volunteer. Stay quiet in discussions. If they can't be invisible and somebody confronts them—*What do you think?*—they shift to compliance, but it's a hollow compliance.

*Oprah*: They answer what they think the other person wants to hear, but they're not engaged in the exchange.

*Dr. Perry*: This is one of the most challenging parts of working with children who have had developmental trauma.

*Oprah*: And it isn't just children. I've seen this behavior in adults. I remember a show we did years ago with Gary Zukav, where a woman explained that after experiencing early sexual abuse, she would sabotage her adult relationships, whether they were happy or not, by removing herself emotionally. She dissociated even though she said she cared deeply about her partner. She'd go through the motions of being in the relationship—compliance—but as you say, it was a hollow compliance. She wasn't really there. But after working with a therapist to create and maintain healthy relationships, she now actively practiced staying present. Gary Zukav validated her feelings by acknowledging that for many people, there is a "terror of being alive." I'll never forget that phrase.

*Dr. Perry*: Interesting that he says that. One of the common behaviors seen with a sensitized dissociative response is cutting. And often someone who cuts will say, "It makes me feel alive—to see my blood. It is soothing."

*Oprah*: Can you please explain the psychology behind cutting? I think I'm not alone in not really understanding how people can be addicted to it.

*Dr. Perry*: Cutting *can* be very confusing from the outside. We've talked about how your stress-response systems can become overly reactive, how anyone experiencing inescapable and unavoidable trauma will dissociate—and how, if the pattern of this trauma is prolonged or extreme, the dissociative systems become sensitized: overactive and overly reactive.

Remember that dissociation releases opioids (enkephalins and endorphins), your own painkillers. If a person without a sensitized dissociative response cuts themselves, their body releases a little bit of these opioids so that they can tolerate the cut; the amount released would be pretty small and proportional to the little cut. But when someone with a sensitized—overly reactive—dissociative response cuts themselves, they release a lot of opioid. It's almost like taking a little hit of heroin or morphine.

*Oprah*: Are you saying it actually feels good? The cut doesn't feel like a cut?

*Dr. Perry*: The opioid "burst" from cutting can actually feel regulating. Soothing. It is rewarding for some. It makes them feel good.

*Oprah*: It doesn't hurt.

*Dr. Perry*: No. In fact, it can become their preferred method of self-regulation.

*Oprah*: I never thought of it that way. So, in order to feel that sense of soothing, you have to be in a dysregulated state. If you're in a regulated state, cutting would hurt, right?

*Dr. Perry*: Right. You have to have a sensitized dissociative response. This usually comes from a history of abuse that was painful, inescapable, and unavoidable—essentially chronic chaos and threat when you were an infant or young child. Or, very often, sexual abuse.

*Oprah*: What's happening to you is inescapable.

*Dr. Perry*: Yes, and then your dissociative neurobiology becomes "sensitized"—overly reactive. And you discover that a reliable way to self-soothe, to ease the pain, is to cut yourself.

*Oprah*: This is fascinating. I've wondered about this for a long time, because I have girls who've come, as we've said before, from difficult, challenged backgrounds. I created OWLAG to give them opportunities, and the trajectory of their lives changed. And yet we had a cutting problem at the school. And each time I was told about it, I wondered how anybody even *knows* to cut themselves. How do they learn to do it? Did they watch someone else? What if the school didn't exist and these same girls were still in their villages or townships? Would they be cutting there? Are people in those villages also cutting?

*Dr. Perry*: That's a really interesting question. If we start with early trauma, little children who have this sensitized response sometimes discover that when they pick at a scab or scratch a mosquito bite— *wow, that feels good*. They begin to learn that self-mutilating can be regulating. But this makes up a fraction of the total group of people who end up cutting. It turns out that many people learn about it from their peers; you can sometimes even track the rates of cutting when a popular TV show talks about it.

Some children will experiment with cutting and say, *No way, this hurts. I'm not doing that anymore.* And others will say, *Wow, that's good.* Just like drugs. A percentage of high-school students will experiment with a drug, but only 18 or 20 percent will end up having trouble with recurrent use. And if you look at the people who go back and use again and again and again, very high percentages of them are the ones who have had developmental adversities. Among the children who don't go back, fewer have had developmental adversities.

*Oprah*: Drugs are a different form of regulation for some people who've experienced trauma.

*Dr. Perry*: So true. There are different maladaptive forms of "self-regulation," but all of them tie into the same basic neurobiology of the stress and reward systems. Some children rock and bang their heads against a wall, for example.

*Oprah*: Yes, I've seen that.

*Dr. Perry*: It has the same effect. And other children will discover that pulling out their hair or their eyebrows gives a little bit of an opiate burst.

*Oprah*: This is so important to understand. I did not realize how this is all tied together.

*Dr. Perry*: Children will find a way to soothe. Making yourself throw up can also cause that opioid burst. So there are eating disorders related to "self-soothing" and not to body image. It's a maladaptive form of soothing.

*Oprah*: This is fascinating, but these behaviors are somewhat extreme. Are there more common coping behaviors?

*Dr. Perry*: Absolutely. And they can develop into personality characteristics that at first are not easy to recognize but may affect how people either avoid or step right into a troublesome situation or interact with challenging people.

*Oprah*: I mentioned earlier that for so much of my life, one of my major personality characteristics was being a people pleaser. It affected everything—my weight, my health, my businesses, my relationships. When you're a victim of abuse and you're taught to be quiet about it, you end up always wanting to please people because you have learned that speaking up will result in punishment. You don't have a concept of how to say no.

*Dr. Perry*: People-pleasing is a classic coping mechanism that is part of the "compliant" behaviors seen with dissociation. But again, it's important to remember that dissociation and self-regulating behaviors that are dissociative are not all bad.

The capacity to control your dissociative capabilities is very powerful. It allows people to be good at reflective cognition. It allows people to have intense focus on a specific task. Hypnosis, flow, being "in the zone"—all of these are examples of the trance state that dissociation allows. People who learn to control when and how they go into a trance state have a gift. I can guarantee you, Oprah, that you're really good at dissociating. It's one of your superpowers.

*Oprah*: Is it?

*Dr. Perry*: Absolutely. Let's start with how you love reading.

*Oprah*: Oh yes, that's true. Books, for me, have always been a way to escape. They were my path to personal freedom. I actually learned to read at the age of three, and once I did, I quickly learned that there was a whole world beyond my grandmother's farm in Mississippi.

*Dr. Perry*: Right. And, you are clearly reflective.

*Oprah*: Oh, very much so.

*Dr. Perry*: And you can go to places in your head and imagine things in the future in ways that a lot of people have a hard time doing. That's dissociation. It's healthy, healing, and productive. This is why people need to be careful about labeling dissociation as a pathology, as a strictly negative behavior. It can be an incredible strength.

But for you, at times, it sounds as if your dissociative adaptations led to you being compliant. You were trying to give people what they wanted.

*Oprah*: Yes, people-pleasing.

*Dr. Perry*: That was your default. Stay under the radar, do what's asked of you, don't give anyone reason to be angry—just give people what they want.

*Oprah*: One hundred percent. Just give people what they want.

*Dr. Perry*: But over time, you have changed. You've dosed yourself away from that overly compliant behavior. You often use the term *intention*—and when you say it, I think "controllable" (see Figure 3). Your life is busy, full of challenges and demands, yet you take that set of stressors and you use boundaries and intention to make the pattern of your life's stress more predictable, controllable, and moderate. That is a healing and resilience-building pattern of stress activation.

*Oprah*: I learned about the power of intention from Gary Zukav. It literally changed everything for me; it's the guiding force in my life. Gary taught me that an intention precedes every thought and every action, and that the outcome of your experiences is determined by your intention going in. It sounds complicated, but really there is nothing I do that doesn't start with my asking myself, *What is my intention in doing this?*

Once I got that, I started to make my decisions based on what I intended, not just on what someone else wanted me to do or what I thought would please them. I had a lot of bullies in my life, but the power of intention helped me create boundaries to do only what I wanted to do because it felt authentic to me. With every decision, big or small, learning to say no has healed me, and intention has saved my life.

But speaking of decisions and choices, I want to turn to a question that baffles so many of us. Why is it that people who are victims of trauma are so often drawn to abusive relationships?

*Dr. Perry*: Let me broaden the question, because it is so important in understanding not just abuse but all behavior. The key point is that all of us tend to gravitate to the familiar, even when the familiar is unhealthy or destructive. We are drawn to what we were raised with.

As we've said before, when we're young and our brain is beginning to make sense of our experiences, it creates our "working model" of the world. The brain organizes around the tone and tension of our first experiences. So if, early on, you have safe, nurturing care, you think that people are inherently good. And, as we also talked about earlier, this worldview makes you project "goodness" onto the people you meet, and that projection of goodness elicits good things in return.

But if as a child you've experienced chaos, threat, or trauma, your brain organizes according to a view that *the world is not safe and people cannot be trusted.* Think about James. He didn't feel "safe" when he was close to people. Intimacy made him feel threatened.

Here is the confusing part: James felt most comfortable when the world was in line with his worldview. Being rejected or treated poorly validated this view. The most destabilizing thing for anyone is to have their core beliefs challenged. As psychologist Virginia Satir puts it, *we feel better with the certainty of misery than the misery of uncertainty.* Good or bad, we are attracted to things that are familiar.

*Oprah*: So if you come from an abusive background, you might be in a relationship with someone who is abusive because it's familiar?

*Dr. Perry*: Yes. In fact, if you get into a relationship with somebody who's not treating you poorly, you may find yourself feeling increasingly uncomfortable. And then, unconsciously, your mind might seek a "predictable" response. You may try to provoke a bit of response. *Maybe I'll do X and it'll piss him off.* If this elicits the behavior you're most familiar with—he gets angry and treats you poorly—it can actually be validating. The worldview has been confirmed. Even though the result is chaos and conflict, it's comforting in the sense that it's familiar.

*Oprah*: I go through this with a lot of my girls at the school. We hand-select young women who are smart and show such promise, but so many were raised in an environment where they did not see or experience what real love looks like or what an expression of real love feels like. For women in their communities, at home and within the family, abuse is systemic. And it goes beyond physical abuse: People don't show up when they say they're going to show up; they don't follow through with what they say they're going to do. Eventually you start to believe that's love. You've been trained. So when one of my girls meets a young man who really is going to respect her, she automatically thinks something's wrong with him. And as you say, she does things to provoke him; in effect, she sabotages the relationship to get him to treat her the way she's accustomed to being treated—to get him to leave. Like Maya Angelou always said, "You teach people how to treat you."

So I really want to know: Is it even possible to fix this, if it's how your brain has developed? And if so, how?

*Dr. Perry*: The good news is that the brain is malleable all through life. We *can* change. But we don't randomly change. To use your favorite word, we can *intentionally* change if we know what needs to be addressed. The key is to recognize the patterns.

*Oprah*: Okay, yes. You start by connecting the dots. But then how do you help people see that this is the same problem showing up? That it's just wearing a different pair of pants? Because that's usually how it works for people. It's the same type of person continually showing up in their life. They might arrive in a different package—it might be a boss or a domineering friend.

I say to my girls, "Look, there's a thread that runs through the course of your life. Look at the kinds of friends you choose, the kinds of personal relationships you have, the boyfriends you are attracted to—and look at what all these people have in common. Then ask yourself how these people make you feel—and which of those feelings trigger feelings you've had before. And then, when you're experiencing these feelings and saying, 'God, I'm so frustrated,' notice whether that person is triggering something that's already there."

*Dr. Perry*: These patterns do run through a person's life—and often through their parents' and grandparents' lives. And without recognizing them, it is very difficult to change. The children and adults we work with are so used to chaos, they actually feel more comfortable when it's chaotic than when it's calm. So when they get into a classroom or a new foster home where people are predictable and consistent and thoughtful, it makes them feel uncomfortable. Little by little, they get more and more uncomfortable until they provoke a predictable response. I have teachers and foster parents tell me, "He almost acts like he *wants* to get punished."

And, to a certain extent, they're right. He is seeking a predictable response from the world. And predictable, for him, means being punished, excluded, minimized. He is looking for evidence that his worldview is accurate: *The world is chaotic. People aren't trustworthy. I don't belong.* He is trying to be kicked out of this class. He is seeking to get kicked out of your home. When we start our work, we try to teach the adults what this behavior really means, and how they can recognize it so they don't reenact it.

Oprah: That's exactly what you told me ten years ago, the very first week my school in South Africa started and I called you on day three.

Dr. Perry: I remember.

Oprah: Girls who had just arrived were suddenly acting out, and we didn't know why. I understood there might be homesickness, but you thought some of them might be having trauma-related issues, even PTSD. You pointed out that no matter how challenging their living conditions had been, we'd taken the girls out of their homes. At home, there were six people sleeping in a bed, and now they're sleeping alone. The sheets are different. The level of comfort is different. The sense of order is different. Everyone at the school is here to love the child—to show support, support, and more support.

Dr. Perry: And this order, stability, and nurturing was a challenge to their worldview. Their brains are going, *What the hell is this?* They're thinking, *I want something familiar.* So they start acting out. They create chaos where there is order, thinking, *I'm going to make something familiar.*

Oprah: I want disorder. I want what is familiar.

Dr. Perry: Exactly. So what you have to do is give these children time and experience. They need patience and understanding and sufficient new experiences to sculpt and shape new views of the world. It takes time to create neural networks with a whole new set of associations. And that is what OWLAG provides for so many of these girls—years of new opportunity; years of cognitively learning new things; and most importantly, years of new relationships, structures, expectations, and new social and emotional lessons. Their worldviews are modified, expanded, clarified, solidified. This takes time, patience, and sometimes therapeutic help.

*Oprah*: But it has to be the right therapy.

*Dr. Perry*: It's interesting—most people think about therapy as something that involves going in and undoing what's happened. But whatever your past experiences created in your brain, the associations exist and you can't just delete them. You can't get rid of the past.

Therapy is more about building *new* associations, making new, healthier default pathways. It is almost as if therapy is taking your two-lane dirt road and building a four-lane freeway alongside it. The old road stays, but you don't use it much anymore. Therapy is building a better alternative, a new default. And that takes repetition, and time; honestly, it works best if someone understands how the brain changes. This is why understanding how trauma impacts our health is essential for everyone.

# CHAPTER 7

# POST-
# TRAUMATIC
# WISDOM

*"Kids are resilient—they'll get over this."*

*I've heard it so many times. Standing with a New York City official in front of the still smoking wreckage of the World Trade Center; sitting with FBI agents and Texas Rangers after the ATF raid on the Branch Davidian compound in Waco; wandering through a blood-splattered apartment with first responders after a shooting witnessed by three young children; talking with district officials after a school shooting—hell, dozens of school shootings. The refrain is all too common: "Good thing children are resilient. They'll be just fine."*

*We often use our belief in another person's "resilience" as an emotional shield. We protect ourselves from the discomfort, confusion, and helplessness we feel in the face of their trauma. It's a kind of looking away; it lets our worldview go unchallenged and lets our life continue with minimal disruption.*

*We see this process play out when an individual is impacted by trauma or grief; often their family, friends, and coworkers begin to orbit a little further out, afraid of the powerful gravitational pull of traumatic pain. As the "check-ins" get fewer, conversations get more superficial, interactions get briefer, and other people "move on" with their lives, the grieving or traumatized person feels increasingly isolated and alone. The emotional bottom does not come in the first weeks following the traumatic event. In those early weeks, family, friends, and community generally mobilize to provide emotional support. Your own physical and mental reserves also help, often through the power of dissociation. But while each person's experience is different, after about six months, you start hitting bottom. And then you drift along the bottom, rising and falling with anniversary reactions, evocative cues, and opportunities to heal. Some people will keep rising; others will drown. None will ever be the same.*

*We see the same rationalization and avoidance in the face of large-scale or community trauma—war, famine, natural disasters, school shootings, the transgenerational impact of slavery. The privileged groups turn their gaze from the pain. In the face of systemic racism, we say, "Look how far they've come"; in the face of cultural genocide, "They need to assimilate"; in the face of trauma, "Isn't it great that they are resilient." It is so easy to create an "other." Us-and-them is deeply ingrained in our neurobiology; it's what makes connectedness a double-edged sword. We are strongly connected to our clan, but not so much to other clans—we compete with them for limited resources.*

*When trauma impacts a group of people or a community, there is an epicenter to the event: the people most impacted by the loss and pain. And there's an immediate mobilization of attention, energy, and resources focused on this epicenter. People rush in to help. But this help is often mistimed, disorganized, and almost always ignorant of trauma. Thousands volunteer their time in the first few weeks; six months later, no one does. After the initial urge to help, the intensity of traumatic loss starts to exhaust and then drive people away. Schools or towns don't want to be identified as being traumatized; they want to be viewed as thriving. People grow tired of hearing about trauma; they want to talk about healing and hope. This is where the well-intentioned efforts to "do something" come in: T-shirts with slogans about strength; teddy bears for still-dazed children. Parents mourning the death of a child are "honored" at a football game. These awkward, kind gestures are part of our struggle to help—and to erase our sense of helplessness.*

*In the wake of trauma, the hardest thing to understand is that nothing and no one can take away the pain. And yet that's exactly what we desperately want to do—because we are social creatures, subject to emotional contagion, and when we're around people who are hurting, we hurt, too. We don't want to hurt. It is hard to sit in the midst of ruined lives and not feel the misery. It helps us regulate to try to undo or negate—to look away from—others' pain.*

*So we make our arbitrary assumptions about people's innate resilience. We make our sweeping declarations that allow us to marginalize traumatized children. We take our focus off the tragedy, move on with our lives, telling ourselves that "they" will be okay. But as we continue to see in our discussions, the impact of trauma doesn't simply fade away.*

*We can help each other heal, but often assumptions about resilience and grit blind us to the healing that leads us down the painful path to wisdom.*

—Dr. Perry

*Oprah*: One of the most thought-provoking things you've ever said is that "children are not born 'resilient,' they are born malleable." Will you explain the difference?

*Dr. Perry*: If you take a Nerf ball and squeeze it, bend it, apply all kinds of force to it, it will, in the end, return to its original ball-like shape. That Nerf ball is resilient. This is the kind of resilience people are talking about when they talk about children being "resilient" in the wake of trauma. They're indulging in the wishful thinking that a child could experience a traumatic stress and somehow, magically, be unaffected. As though the child would be able to return to their prior level of emotional, physical, social, and cognitive health, unchanged. But as we've spent this whole book discussing, that is simply not the way it works. We are always changing. We change from all of our experiences, good and bad. This is because our brain is changeable—malleable. It's *always* changing.

Think about a metal hanger. Let's say you need to fish something out of a drain, and the hanger is your best tool. You apply force to bend it into the shape you want. The hanger is malleable. When the job is done, you can try to bend it back to its original shape, but even if you're a champion hanger-bender, you won't get it to exactly what it was. And there will be weaknesses in the places where you bent it. And if you were to keep bending and restoring it in the same places, the hanger would ultimately break.

Now, we talked earlier about resilience, and it is true that both children and adults can "demonstrate resilience," as we say in our field, in the face of a challenge or even trauma. You can demonstrate resilience and, as we've said, you can build resilience. But it's not resilience in the Nerf-ball sense. And it's not an automatic property of childhood. The capacity to get back to "baseline" after a trauma is influenced by many factors, primarily your connectedness.

*Oprah*: So you're saying that no matter what age you are, no one emerges from a trauma unscathed? And that it's impossible to go back to being "the same" once a trauma has occurred?

*Dr. Perry*: To a degree, yes, that is what I am saying. Again, though, to clarify: The concept of resilience *is* used in our field. But if you look carefully at our biology after a traumatic experience—all the way down to the way genes are expressed—trauma will change everyone in some way.

And these changes will be there even if they don't result in any apparent "real life" problems for the person, even if the person demonstrates resilience. A child may continue to do just as well in school, for example, but it may take much more energy and effort. Or we may find that a child is able to return to his previous level of emotional functioning, but changes in his neuroendocrine system may make him more likely to develop diabetes. This is, in essence, what the ACE studies have demonstrated: Adversity impacts the developing child. Period. What that impact will be, when it may manifest, how it may be "buffered"—we can't always say. But developmental trauma will always influence our body and brain.

*Oprah*: If you look at the brain of a traumatized child, will it look different?

*Dr. Perry*: Our current brain-imaging techniques are pretty sophisticated, but they're not yet sensitive enough to scan an individual child and say with confidence, for example, "This underactivity in the prefrontal cortex is from abuse." What we do know is that if you compare a group of children who've experienced no abuse with a group of children who've experienced similar timing and type of abuse, there will be statistically significant differences in the size of some areas of the brain, some differences in "connections," some differences in "activity." But the complexities of development, the brain, and the nature of trauma make neuroimaging studies very difficult to interpret.

*Oprah*: So if you were to look at the brain of a three-year-old who was nurtured and supported, and the brain of a three-year-old who was neglected and abused, could you see a difference?

*Dr. Perry*: Again, this is very complex, but if the neglect were in the "total global neglect" category, yes. Using the right imaging techniques, you can see differences. But again, these are really difficult to interpret.

The actual best indicators of change in the brain following trauma or neglect are "functional" changes: Is the child impulsive or inattentive? Do they have speech and language problems or fine-motor-control issues? Are they depressed or anxious? Do they have a hard time learning? Can they form and maintain healthy relationships? All of these things are much better indicators of changes in the brain than brain scans are.

Now, brain scans *have* shown us that each of us has a unique brain—which, considering everything we've been talking about, is not surprising. And because each of us has a unique brain, we will experience stress, distress, and trauma in a somewhat unique way. Two people who experience the same traumatic event can respond differently—and recover differently. When a person is able to "recover" emotionally—returning to a pre-trauma level of functioning—we refer to that as demonstrating resilience. And the capacity to do that is malleable. In other words, the ability to cope with stress, distress, and trauma is changeable. It's something that we can help build in people. You can make your coping machinery stronger and more effective.

*Oprah*: When I was a child, we used the term *weathering*. We didn't have a word for the kind of trauma so many African Americans endured, so we said we "weathered." The church was a big part of how we got through. We weathered together.

*Dr. Perry*: You are identifying such a central aspect of building resilience. Your connectedness to other people is so key to buffering any current stressor—and to healing from past trauma. Being with people who are present, supportive, and nurturing. Belonging.

Of course, other factors also impact a person's capacity to demonstrate resilience. Some of the most important are related to the sensitivity of your stress-response systems. Anything that makes those systems more reactive or sensitive will make you more vulnerable. This could include genetic factors, intrauterine exposure to alcohol, a history of attachment problems, or previous trauma.

Let's go back to the start of our conversation, back to our core regulatory networks. The CRNs comprise a set of very important neural networks that collectively reach every part of your body and brain. We know that when these systems are well-organized, flexible, and "strong," we have the capacity to cope with all manner of stressors (Figures 2 and 3).

We also know that controllable, predictable, and moderate challenges can make the CRNs even stronger. Our stress-response capabilities expand when they get "practice." So if a child has had the opportunity to have predictable, moderate challenges as they grow up, they will be more capable of demonstrating resilience in the face of a challenge.

. The very start of this process is when the newborn is hungry, thirsty, or cold, and the attentive, attuned caregiver meets their needs. Later, they'll crawl away from the safety of their parent and start exploring the world; because this is novel, it will activate their stress response—but only moderately. When it becomes too much, they'll crawl back to the "safe base." This process—leave the safe, explore the new, return to the safe—will continue thousands of times for the toddler and young child. And through these little challenges, they build the capacity to demonstrate resilience in the face of unexpected stress.

All development involves being exposed to novelty, which in turn activates our stress response. With a safe and stable relational foundation, thousands of moderate doses of stress help create flexible stress-response capabilities. Every school year, meeting new classmates and a new teacher and studying new content provides moderate, predictable stressors. Participating in sports, music, drama, and other activities creates more opportunities for the controllable, predictable stress that helps build resilience.

And through all of this, *relationships* are absolutely key. For the infant, the relationship with primary caregivers is the foundation of their capacity for all future relationships. It is in the context of nurturing and caring relationships that the child can meet a challenge; in the face of any new challenge, an adult can model, encourage, and provide a helping hand. And the relational reward—the smile, word of encouragement, congratulations for progress during and after the challenge—motivates the child, which leads to repetition and mastery. A child without these relational supports will not have as many developmental successes.

It's really important to note that the supportive parent, teacher, or coach also helps provide the proper "dosing" of challenge for the child. Challenges should fit the child's developmental stage, because impossible challenges set up children to fail. A child who has not yet learned to multiply cannot be expected to learn algebra; a child who has just learned to write words cannot be expected to write full paragraphs. It's a Goldilocks situation. Just as the challenge shouldn't be too big, it also shouldn't be too small; it has to be novel enough to cause the child to leave the comfort zone of their known experiences and already-mastered skills. If the challenge is going to build resilience, it has to be moderate—just right.

Finding the "just right" is a major issue with children who have had trauma. Remember, they frequently live in a persistent state of fear. And fear shuts down parts of the cortex—the thinking part of the brain. In a classroom, what may seem to be a moderate, developmentally appropriate challenge for many children may be an overwhelming demand on a child with a sensitized stress response (see Figure 5).

*Oprah:* So children need challenges to build resilience, but the stress of the challenges has to be just right, and the scaffolding of support has to be in place or the child can get dysregulated and fail. In which case, rather than building confidence and resilience, you risk eroding self-esteem or worse.

*Dr. Perry:* That's right. You need moderate activation of your stress response. You can't become a good athlete unless you stress and challenge your cardiovascular system and your muscles, but you have to do it in a way that's predictable and moderate. Otherwise, you risk injury.

*Oprah:* And you can't become a healthy human being unless you've had some challenges that allow you to build resilience and empathy.

*Dr. Perry:* Yes. Healthy development involves a series of challenges and exposure to new things. And failure is an important part of the process. We try, we fall, we get up, we try again. And again. All developmental success comes after failure, and typically many failures will occur before mastery is achieved. The key is to have challenges that are achievable—close enough to your current capabilities that you will succeed with some encouragement, practice, and repetition.

A child in an environment where they feel loved and safe will choose to leave their comfort zone. Safe and familiar is "boring"; a safe and stable child is a curious child—they want to explore new things. A child who feels unsafe, however, won't want this. It's an essential rule of healthy development: A sense of safety and stability provides a foundation for healthy growth.

*Oprah*: The process you're describing will be very different if the child is in a home where there's been nothing but chaos or a lack of dependability. I'm thinking of all the people we encounter who are ready to fight the minute you say anything they feel is critical or confrontational; the slightest thing, and they're ready to blow.

*Dr. Perry*: Yes, this might be someone with a sensitized stress-response system. Our brain processes incoming sensory input from the bottom up (see Figures 2 and 10), and if someone has a life with chaotic, uncontrollable, or extreme and prolonged stress, particularly early in life, they're more likely to act before thinking. Their cortex is not as active, and reactivity in the lower areas of the brain becomes more dominant.

It's very difficult to meaningfully connect with or get through to someone who is not regulated. And it's nearly impossible to reason with them. This is why telling someone who is dysregulated to "calm down" never works.

*Oprah*: It just makes them angrier.

*Dr. Perry*: Of course. When someone is very upset, words themselves are not very effective. The tone and rhythm of the voice probably has more impact than the actual words.

*Oprah*: So you want to be present with them?

*Dr. Perry*: Yes, it's best if you can simply be present. If you do use words, it's best to restate what they're saying; this is called *reflective listening*. You can't talk someone out of feeling angry, sad, or frustrated, but you can be a sponge and absorb their emotional intensity. If you stay regulated, ultimately they will "catch" your calm. It also helps to use some form of rhythmic regulating activity to keep yourself regulated while you're doing this—like taking a walk, kicking a ball back and forth, shooting some baskets, coloring side-by-side; there are dozens of rhythmic ways to help us regulate.

*Oprah*: Because doing things with movement and rhythm offers a more connected way of communicating.

*Dr. Perry*: As we discussed, rhythm is so important, and it's often overlooked as a therapeutic tool. I remember a time I was listening to Mike Roseman, the Korean War veteran we met in Chapter 1. He was talking about his weekend. I say "listening," but in fact I was partially listening, partially mind-wandering. I felt like I had heard this same thing a dozen times. "I slept like a baby on Saturday night, slept all night long. Felt really good on Sunday. Then I had a terrible night again last night." Then something clicked. I *had* heard this a dozen times! Every Monday Mike said the same thing about Saturday night.

I looked at him sheepishly. "What did you say you did this weekend?"

He said, "We went to dinner and then to a dance club."

"And what do you do at the dance club?"

He looked at me and raised his eyebrows.

"Oh. You dance, right? But how much? Do you dance for hours or just for one or two songs? Waltz? Hip-hop?"

"They play all kinds of music, but mostly it's swing, a little rock and roll sometimes. I pretty much dance on and off for three hours."

"And last week you told me you fell asleep at physical therapy when they gave you a massage at the end of the session, right?"

"Yes."

Thinking about this helped me begin to piece together the regulating potential of patterned, repetitive activity like dancing or massage. As you recall, Mike Roseman had PTSD. His stress-response system, including his CRNs, was overactive and overly reactive. That made it hard for him to fall asleep. And when he did, his sensitized stress-response system made it hard to transition smoothly through the various stages of sleep. As a result, he was a very light sleeper, typically waking after a few hours; many nights he would doze for only a few minutes before startling awake at the slightest noise. He was always exhausted. But now he was telling me that he had a long, deep, refreshing sleep after hours of dancing and that he fell asleep in minutes when he was getting a massage.

From that point forward, a major component of Mike's therapy was "physical therapy." Several times a week he would get massages for his "bad back." I encouraged him to dance in smaller doses all week long, and to walk. He started walking all over town. A month or so after creating a more structured schedule of rhythmic activities, he began sleeping much better. And his other post-traumatic symptoms started to be less intrusive.

*Oprah*: It's incredible that something as simple as walking can have that effect. Walking is very regulating for me.

*Dr. Perry*: And it's especially regulating if you can walk in nature. The sensory elements of the natural world bathe us with their own regulating rhythms.

Let's keep talking about how you can help a dysregulated person feel more regulated. Instead of saying, *Hey, tell me what you're thinking about,* you need to let them control when and how much they're going to talk about what's upsetting them. If you give a person that control and help them feel safe, in their own time they will be more capable of talking.

*Oprah*: Yes! I remember the first time I interviewed Elizabeth Smart's parents. You may recall that Elizabeth was taken at knifepoint from her home in Salt Lake City at the age of fourteen and was held captive for more than nine months. When I interviewed her parents after she was recovered, I asked, "What has she said about it? What have you talked about?" And they told me she hadn't said anything yet. At the time, I was surprised, but I now understand that they were waiting for her. In her own time. In her own way. Because, as you're saying, if *you* control when and how much a traumatized person talks, it can be retraumatizing rather than healing.

*Dr. Perry*: Exactly. We want to provide therapeutic, healing interactions. Moderate, controllable, and predictable interactions. Remember the way you described talking with Gayle? And the little boy who told the checkout clerk that his mother was dead? Controlling when, how much, and which aspect of a traumatic event they share allows a person to create their own therapeutic pattern of recovery. No one knows what a moderate dose of revisiting a trauma memory is better than the actual traumatized person. For the little boy in the grocery store, it was literally only seconds long.

We've talked a lot about patterns of stress activation that create "sensitization," which is essentially the opposite of resilience. But when we activate trauma memories and our stress-response systems in ways that offer controllability and predictability, we can begin to heal a sensitized system. Healing takes place when there are dozens of therapeutic moments available each day for the person to control, revisiting and reworking their traumatic experience.

When you have friends, family, and other healthy people in your life, you have a natural healing environment. We heal best in community. Creating a network—a village, whatever you want to call it—gives you opportunities to revisit trauma in moderate, controllable doses. That pattern of stress activation will ultimately lead to a more regulated stress-reactivity curve (see Figure 5). So the traumatized person with a sensitized stress response can become "neurotypical"—less sensitized, less vulnerable. In fact, they can ultimately develop the capacity to demonstrate resilience.

The journey from *traumatized* to *typical* to *resilient* helps create a unique strength and perspective. That journey can create post-traumatic wisdom.

For thousands and thousands of years, humans lived in small intergenerational groups. There were no mental health clinics—but there was plenty of trauma. I assume that many of our ancestors experienced post-traumatic problems: anxiety, depression, sleep disruptions. But I also assume that they experienced healing. Our species could not have survived if a majority of our traumatized ancestors lost their capacity to function well. The pillars of traditional healing were 1) connection to clan and the natural world; 2) regulating rhythm through dance, drumming, and song; 3) a set of beliefs, values, and stories that brought meaning to even senseless, random trauma; and 4) on occasion, natural hallucinogens or other plant-derived substances used to facilitate healing with the guidance of a healer or elder.

It is not surprising that today's best practices in trauma treatment are basically versions of these four things. Unfortunately, few modern approaches use all four of the options well. The medical model overfocuses on psychopharmacology (4) and cognitive behavioral approaches (3). It greatly undervalues the power of connectedness (1) and rhythm (2).

I once worked with a four-year-old girl named Ally. She had witnessed the death of her mother at the hands of her father, who then committed suicide. Ally lived in a very close-knit community, and after the traumatic loss of her parents, she moved in with one of her aunts. There were easily thirty cousins, aunts, uncles, and grandparents living in the community. And they were always together for birthdays, holidays, family events. Ally was an active part of her church, played sports, and had a very supportive elementary school with "trauma-sensitive" teachers. Part of our work with her was educating the adults in her life—including her teachers—about trauma. In the first weeks after Ally was found, we saw her about three times a week. Within a month, it was down to once a week. After the first-year anniversary, we needed to see her only once a month. Six months later, we told her aunt to simply reach out if there were any questions or problems. The last I heard about Ally was that she'd been elected class president at her middle school, was active in sports and her church, and was doing very well in school. She and her aunt reported no significant symptoms. Of course there was sadness on occasions, but Ally was a positive, happy, engaging girl. The scars remained, but she was weathering well. And she was a wise soul. She had developed post-traumatic wisdom.

*Oprah*: Post-traumatic wisdom. I love that. Ally's experience has a positive outcome. So isn't that an example of a child being resilient?

*Dr. Perry*: Absolutely. But not because she was born resilient. Ally was able to show resilience in the face of tragedy due to the quality of loving relationships earlier in her life. Resilience is a capability that can wax and wane, not a permanent, innate trait. If Ally hadn't had a safe, stable, and nurturing family, an understanding teacher, or her strong faith, her ability to "bounce back" would have quickly drained away. Her ability to heal and continue to demonstrate resilience was related to ongoing safe and stable relationships through which she could "make sense" of horror and put it in the context of her beliefs. Even the most seemingly resilient people can be drained by relational poverty and ongoing stress, distress, and trauma.

*Oprah*: Ally's story, and the way you described the healing power of the intergenerational clans from thousands of years ago, makes me think of growing up in Kosciusko, Mississippi, and how the church was the center point of our life. Every week I'd be there for Sunday school followed by the eleven o'clock service. We'd go home, and my grandmother would cook before we returned for another service at three o'clock, then Baptist Union training at five or six. On Wednesday nights we'd go for a prayer service and choir rehearsal. At three and a half years old, I was speaking in front of the congregation. The hours I spent in that little white church by the red dirt road certainly formed the spiritual foundation for my life.

Later, when I was living in Nashville with my father, I accepted a job as a reporter at a television station in Baltimore. As I was preparing to leave my family and the life I knew, my father's advice to me was "Find a church home." At the time, I thought it was because he wanted to make sure I kept Jesus in my life. Looking back now, though, as we talk about the healing power of relationships, I realize it wasn't just about finding a place of worship—it was about finding a community, and discovering true, lasting connection in a new city.

In those days, church was everything: your counselor, your nurturer, your comforter, your refuge. The idea of going to therapy wasn't even discussed; if you needed help, you went to church. As I said, we weathered together. It was your church family that made sure you had a place to go for Sunday dinner. They were the ones who visited you when you were sick or passed around the collection plate if you couldn't put food on the table.

The church was even where we created that healing sense of rhythm. Our music connected and lifted us.

For many people, church isn't their thing, but everyone needs people who can listen, be present, and make them feel heard and seen. And as we're talking, I see that a key to healing from trauma is finding your "church home"—your people, your community. This can help build resilience, post-traumatic healing, and ultimately post-traumatic wisdom. It can help you become wise.

*Dr. Perry*: It is impossible to be truly wise without some real-life hardship. And we cannot develop post-traumatic wisdom without weathering and, most importantly, as you point out, weathering together.

*Oprah*: Social connection builds resilience, and resilience helps create post-traumatic wisdom, and that wisdom leads to hope. Hope for you and hope for others witnessing and participating in your healing, hope for your community.

*Dr. Perry*: Absolutely. A healthy community is a healing community, and a healing community is full of hope because it has seen its own people weather—survive and thrive.

The first time I saw how a healing community can work was almost thirty years ago. This experience completely shifted the way I think about therapeutics; I started to understand that most therapeutic experience—most healing—happens outside of formal therapy. Most healing happens in *community*.

In February of 1993, the Bureau of Alcohol, Tobacco, Firearms, and Explosives (ATF) attempted a raid on David Koresh's Branch Davidian compound in Waco, Texas. Four ATF members and six Davidians were killed in the raid. Over the next three days, the FBI negotiated the release of twenty-one of the children in the compound. Then these releases stopped, and a fifty-one-day siege ensued. It ended with an FBI assault that precipitated a Davidian-lit fire, which killed seventy-six Davidians, including the remaining twenty-five children.

Several days after the initial ATF raid, I was asked by officials of the State of Texas to lead a clinical team to care for the released Davidian children. They were all housed in a single large cottage on the Methodist Home campus in Waco. They ranged in age from three to thirteen, a mix of boys and girls. They had been in an hours-long firefight and had seen members of their community die. Each of them had been separated from family and handed over to complete strangers, usually armed FBI agents in SWAT gear.

In the days before we took over, the children experienced chaos. Each day was unpredictable, and each child interacted with dozens of strange people, some of them armed. While growing up, the children had been indoctrinated to believe that all non-Davidians were "Babylonians" intent on destroying David Koresh and all of his followers. So here were these children, torn away from everything they knew, being cared for by people they believed would kill them. Bottom line, this was a group of acutely traumatized children.

In the first days we worked with them, the children exhibited various acute post-traumatic effects; for example, as a group, the average resting heart rate was 132, whereas normal would have been less than 90. There was some pressure to "do therapy" with these children. But I knew that talking with dysregulated children was not going to be effective. I felt our first task should be to bring structure and predictability to their day.

We started to make the uncontrollable and unpredictable more controllable and predictable. I limited unnecessary access to the children—no more new adults. We had group meetings in the morning, to outline the day, and in the evening, to review the day; at the meetings, the children had opportunities to ask questions. We had play, quiet time, and meals—always at the same time. And we gave the children multiple opportunities to make choices—about what they ate, what they played with, how they spent their quiet time.

Each day after the children went to bed, our team would meet. We would talk about each child, and any member of the team who'd had any interaction with that child was asked to describe it. I logged these brief interactions on a spreadsheet, hour by hour. Many were brief therapeutic moments: A child would ask, "What do you think will happen to my mom?"—then listen to a reassuring comment and drift back to play. The children were controlling when and how they talked about the traumatic events they'd experienced. They were also seeking safe, stable, and physically regulating interactions. "Push me on the swing." "Let's draw." As I added up the interactions, I saw that despite no formal "therapy" sessions, the children were getting over two hours of therapeutic interaction each day. By the end of three weeks with our team, the children were much more regulated; the group heart rate had dropped below 100, into the normal range. They were more interactive and talkative, and the therapeutic interactions became more verbal.

One of the most important observations was that these children needed different kinds of therapeutic interaction at different times. They knew this even better than we did. A child who wanted quiet nurturing interactions would seek out one of our staff who was a really good listener and able to sit quietly without talking—not easy for most adults. When this same child wanted to play, they'd seek out a member of our team who was younger and more playful; when they wanted reassurance from an authority figure, they'd come to me. Each of us had a unique set of personality characteristics, and at any given moment our particular strength might be just what one of the children needed. No one person, no single therapist could be all things for all the children, who were each at different stages of development and in different states of regulation. Our clinical structure at Waco reminded me of the importance of developmental "diversity" for children.

Think of the diversity within a small multifamily, multigenerational clan. Children growing up had numerous adults and older children who could model, teach, nurture, discipline, and care for them. Each person in the clan had a unique set of strengths—the right person at the right time. No single person was expected to provide all of the emotional, social, physical, or cognitive needs of the developing child.

This is incredibly unlike our modern world. We expect a single working mother to be the one to throw the baseball with her eight-year-old, rock the newborn, read to the three-year-old, and, by the way, cook a nutritious meal, help with homework, do the laundry, get everyone to bed, then wake up and get them all ready for childcare and school so she can go work all day, only to rush home to do it all again. All alone.

*Oprah*: She needs people to step up—people who support her, give her some breaks, step in and do some of those things with her children. We're not meant to be isolated and alone. We're actually meant to work together. So when a single mom is living on a limited income, trying to manage four children, trying to be mother and father, and she feels overwhelmed or feels like it's impossible to do it all—it's because it *is* impossible.

*Dr. Perry*: It's such an unfair expectation of our society. No other society in the history of this planet has ever asked a single adult to provide the physical, social, emotional, and material needs of multiple children by themselves.

*Oprah*: You're not meant to raise children isolated and alone.

*Dr. Perry*: Absolutely not. We are meant to distribute caregiving among the many adults in our "band"—our community. In a typical hunter-gatherer clan, for every child under six there were four developmentally more mature individuals who could model, discipline, nurture, and instruct the child. That is a 4:1 ratio: four developmentally mature individuals for each child under six. We now think that one caregiver for four young children (1:4) is "enriched." That is 1/16th of what our developing social brain is looking for. That is relational poverty.

*Oprah*: It makes me want to weep for all the single parents out there who are doing it every day and breaking their backs, their spirits, and not even able to take care of themselves. It also makes me think of my mother differently. She did the best she could and was often too tired to do any better.

*Dr. Perry*: And single parents, like your mother, often end up feeling like they are inadequate—that there is something wrong with them, that they aren't enough. When really, it's the modern world that's not enough.

A strong connection to community is as important today as it was thousands of years ago. The tragedy of the modern world is that community like this is harder and harder to find. Not everybody has friends like Gayle. Fewer people are active in their community of faith. Not everybody feels like they belong. There is a direct relationship between a person's degree of social isolation and their risk for physical and mental health problems.

But when you do have connectedness—your "church home"—you have built-in buffers for whatever stress or distress you experience.

*Oprah*: We do belong. We are enough. But it's hard to see that in our current world.

*Dr. Perry*: Imagine that your annual review at work goes badly. Your supervisor gives you some negative feedback. You feel really upset. You keep thinking about it. You run it through your head again and again. You go back and talk to one of your colleagues. "Can you believe he said that? I don't think that's true!" And your colleague listens and reassures you: "No, that's not true. He's full of it." You feel soothed for a bit. Then you call another colleague and run it by her. And you go home and you go over it with your partner.

You've engaged in three, four, or five "doses" where you controlled how and when you talked about the distressing feedback. As your perspective is heard, you become regulated, reassured. The next day, you feel better. You have created a controllable and moderate revisiting of the distressing review, and that has changed your reaction to it. It is no longer as distressing. Originally you were dysregulated, you shut down the "rational" part of your head, distorted the comments, magnified them. But now you can reflect more accurately on the feedback, and maybe see some truth in the comments. That wasn't possible until you could use your many relational interactions to revisit and regulate.

When we have a community, we can do this kind of dosing to regulate any stressful or distressing experience. We can build and demonstrate resilience. We do so all the time. But imagine someone without the relationships that would allow this kind of relational regulation. For someone with relational poverty, these stressful experiences are magnified by the echo chamber of their own head. Stress becomes distress. And distressing experiences become sensitizing, resulting in the same physical and mental effects as trauma.

This is the challenge for our modern world. How can we create community when we are so mobile, so screened up, so disconnected? It's a major challenge for creating a healthy future. How can we ensure connectedness, and a sense of safety and belonging for everyone?

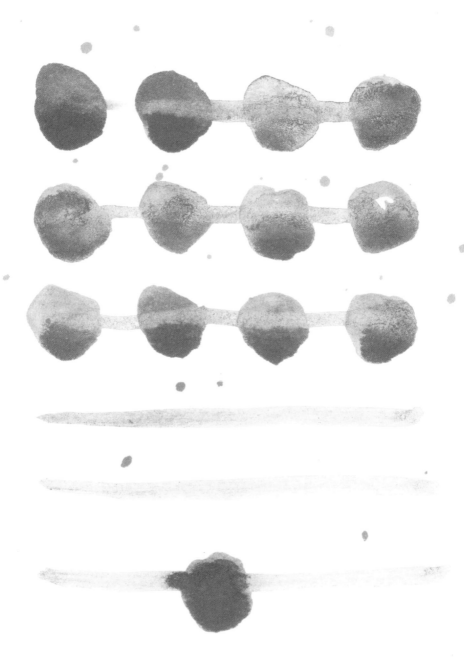

# CHAPTER 8

# OUR BRAINS, OUR BIASES, OUR SYSTEMS

In 2015, I interviewed a man named Shaka Senghor for my show Super Soul Sunday. At the age of nineteen, Shaka had been convicted of second-degree murder. He served nineteen years in prison, including a total of seven years in solitary confinement. At the beginning of his sentence, Shaka was angry and violent, and quickly sank into a system that had no interest in preparing him for his eventual return to the outside world. But after six years behind bars, something shifted, and Shaka began to transform. In his five-by-seven cell, he started meditating, reading, journaling—and writing what would eventually become his bestselling memoir, Writing My Wrongs.

When I first saw a photo of Shaka on the cover of his book, I was skeptical. What could this tattooed, dreadlocked convicted killer teach me?

Our conversation was one of the best I've ever experienced.

As his story unfolded over the course of our two and a half hours together, so did my understanding—of what it means to fall short, what it means to go astray, and what it truly means to be shaped by your environment.

Shaka, born James White, grew up in a middle-class family in Detroit. His father, a member of the Air Force Reserves, worked for the state of Michigan. His mother stayed at home with James and his five siblings. As a young boy, James was a straight-A student with dreams of becoming a doctor.

From the outside, the Whites looked like the ideal American family. But Shaka says for as long as he can remember, his mother had an explosive temper and took out her rage on her children.

"Did you feel loved growing up?" I asked him.

"I was told, 'I do this because I love you,'" he said. "But it was always a whupping or a punishment." I connected to this immediately.

Shaka recalled coming home from school one day when he was nine, thrilled to have gotten an A+ on a test and hoping his mother would share his joy. Instead, she threw a pot at him so furiously, it cracked the tiles on the kitchen wall behind him.

*I asked if he ever found out what she was upset about.*

*"I never knew," he said. "My mother was upset often."*

*As I listened, my heart broke for Shaka and the millions of people who as children regularly experienced paralyzing fear at home. The tragedy isn't just what that fear felt like in the moment—it's that they learned to bury the emotion and accept the behavior.*

*In addition to his mother's physical abuse, Shaka says the last five years of his parents' marriage were unstable. He was devastated by their separations and rejoiced at their reunions, gutted and lifted each time the cycle repeated. When they finally divorced, Shaka, tired of being betrayed by the people he loved most, says he built an emotional wall and sought protection and acceptance from the streets. He began acting out: getting in fights, refusing to do school-work, running away from home.*

*What struck me most about Shaka's story is that at no time during this change—from straight-A student to street kid—did anyone ask, "What happened to you? Why are you behaving this way?" Not one adult seemed to notice or care that this young boy had completely lost his way.*

*By age fourteen, Shaka was selling drugs, breaking into houses, and shoplifting. After being shot at seventeen, he began carrying a gun with him at all times. He was in a culture and environment that perpetuated the idea that a young man's worth was defined by hav-ing money, attention, and a reputation as "the bad guy."*

*"In that space, I felt accepted," Shaka told me. "I was around other broken, fragile young males, and we banded together around our brokenness. I thought,* This is support. This is love. This is 'I got your back no matter what.'"

*"But weren't you the smart one who wanted to be a doctor?" I asked. "Why did you want to be a doctor?"*

*He paused—for twenty-three seconds—an eternity in TV time. I could tell he'd never really thought about this before. "My mother* was always nice when she took me to the doctor," he finally said. He paused again. His eyes welled. "I guess I imagined if I became a doctor, she would be nice to me." It was a deeply moving moment of realization for both of us: a young man, confused and rejected by those who were charged with raising him, simply seeking his mother's validation and love.

When he was nineteen, Shaka's dangerous life choices came to a head. One night, on his way home from a party, he started arguing with a man named David. In the middle of the fight, Shaka grabbed his gun and pulled the trigger and shot David dead.

In prison, Shaka found an environment he was familiar with, one where violence and domination reigned. He repeatedly landed himself in solitary confinement, for everything from assaulting prison guards to trying to escape.

What finally broke him open was a letter from his son.

"Dear Dad," the letter read. "My mother told me you was in prison for murder. Dear Dad, don't murder anymore. Jesus watches what you do. Pray to him, and he'll forgive your sins."

"That part is what just shattered everything," Shaka told me. "I thought, I refuse for that to be the legacy for my child. That was the moment that I decided that I would never go back to the darkness and that I had to find my light. And that I owed it to him to find my light."

Since Shaka's release from prison in 2010, he's been a vocal advocate for criminal-justice reform. He speaks to young people across the country, sharing his story and encouraging young men to avoid life on the streets. He's taught classes at the University of Michigan and is a fellow of the MIT Media Lab. At the heart of his work is the belief that people should not be defined by their past mistakes, and that redemption is possible.

Most people who are in the process of excavating the reasons they do what they do are met at some point with resistance. "You're blaming the past." "Your past is not an excuse."

*This is true. Your past is not an excuse. But it is an* explanation—
*offering insight into the questions so many of us ask ourselves:* Why
do I behave the way I behave? Why do I feel the way I do? *For me,
there is no doubt that our strengths, vulnerabilities, and unique
responses are an expression of what happened to us.*

*Very often, "what happened" takes years to reveal itself. It takes
courage to confront our actions, peel back the layers of trauma in
our lives, and expose the raw truth of our past. But this is where
healing begins.*

—Oprah

*Oprah*: When we first started talking about trauma, over thirty years ago, not many people were aware of its impact on so many aspects of life. Have things changed? When you look at schools, the health-care system, the criminal-justice system—really everywhere you look—there are people impacted by trauma who are still misunderstood, and sometimes retraumatized, by the very systems that should be helping them.

*Dr. Perry*: That is the heartbreaking truth. It takes a long time to change people—and even longer to change systems. I *am* optimistic, though. Many positive changes are underway. Many more people are aware of how pervasive trauma is. More people understand that trauma can influence our health. But we do have a long way to go. We need more professionals and organizations to change the way they "do business" to help address the impact of trauma.

*Oprah*: You're talking about trauma-informed care?

*Dr. Perry*: Yes and no. As you know, I'm not a fan of that term. I'm impressed by what is happening in many places attempting to implement "trauma-informed care," but I think the language is getting in the way of progress. Let me explain why.

As we have been discussing, the complexities of trauma impact all of our systems, from maternal-child health to child welfare to education, law enforcement, mental health, and more. Each of these systems is a world unto itself, with its own professionals, its own attitudes, its own language. We've talked about how individual people develop their unique "worldview"—well, the same thing happens with systems and organizations; they develop a dominant perspective. In the past, most of these perspectives have not included any significant understanding of development, stress, or trauma—or interrelated issues that can cause distress or trauma such as implicit bias, racism, and misogyny. But with so much new research emerging about these areas and these issues, it's become clear that our systems can't ignore them. And as each system has grappled with what "trauma-informed" means, they've used their own particular lens— their own view of the world.

The result is that defining the term has been a challenge. Like the word *trauma,* it's been used by many different people and groups in many different ways. It may take some time to sort this out.

The term trauma-informed care—or TIC—emerged back in 2001 to encourage mental health and child-welfare systems to recognize that trauma was an important but misunderstood factor in the lives of the people these systems were serving.

Over time, many groups started to use the term, with minimal definition or clarity. Organizations would have a three-hour seminar and declare themselves "trauma-informed." Cities gave themselves the label; even countries aspired to becoming the "first trauma-informed nation." All of this was confusing. What constitutes a "trauma-informed" city, anyway? Buzzwords abounded, but they were rarely connected to concrete implementation plans or changes in services, programs, or policy. TIC "training" became a cottage industry, with hundreds of organizations and "experts" willing to take your money to ensure that you and your organization were trauma-informed. The quality of this training was, as you might expect, highly inconsistent.

In response to this chaotic beginning, scores of countries, states, professional organizations, interdisciplinary committees, and professional teams worked to define and implement TIC. Unfortunately, these disjointed efforts further complicated things. As one committee concluded: *"Despite years of work in the field, there is not a common definition of TIC."*

Dozens of versions of the crucial "elements," "principles," "pillars," "ingredients," "assumptions," "components," "domains," and "guidelines" of TIC have emerged. But while there are some consistent concepts, the variability is head-spinning.

The result is that you never know which version of TIC someone is thinking of when they use the term. This is why, when I'm talking about trauma practice, programs, or policy, I always try to describe the specific concepts, content, or objective—rather than use the term TIC.

Having said all this, I do think that these efforts are really important. And that progress is being made. All of these organizations are teaching about trauma, advocating for increased public awareness, and supporting research to learn more; many are evaluating and promoting promising interventions. In 1989, the National Center for PTSD was formed within the Department of Veterans Affairs (VA) to study trauma and support veterans impacted by, mostly, combat-related trauma. In 2000, the National Center for Child Traumatic Stress was formed. It wasn't until 2018 that the branches of the CDC and SAMHSA dedicated to studying trauma came up with their seven principles of TIC, which I suspect will continue to evolve as the field grows up.

It's easy to forget how young traumatology—the study of trauma—is. And developmental traumatology, as a discipline, is even younger. Right now, organizations and systems are just starting to grapple with the very issues we've been discussing in this book. And grapple they must, because trauma permeates all aspects of life; it echoes through the generations, across families, communities, institutions, cultures, and societies, and it does so in very complex ways. Trauma can impact our genes, white blood cells, heart, gut, lungs, and brain, our thinking, feeling, behaving, parenting, teaching, coaching, consuming, creating, prescribing, arresting, sentencing. I could go on.

So, depending upon your perspective—your worldview—and your own history of trauma and loss, you will have some unique version of "trauma-informed."

*Oprah*: But in essence, it's approaching people with the awareness that "what happened to you" is important, that it influences your behavior and your health. And then using that awareness to act accordingly and respond appropriately—whether you're a parent, teacher, friend, therapist, doctor, police officer, judge.

*Dr. Perry*: Yes, absolutely. That captures, as well as any other brief statement, the essence of "trauma-informed." The "act accordingly" part is so important. It's one thing to be aware that trauma can result in certain behaviors and problems. It's another thing to ask, "What do we do now?"

How do we create opportunities for healing within our systems? How can we avoid repeating unpredictable, uncontrollable stressors that will exacerbate the effects of trauma? How do we make sure we don't "retraumatize" someone by unintentionally continuing the marginalizing, dehumanizing experiences that gave rise to the very problems we're supposed to be addressing?

I believe that if you don't recognize the built-in biases in yourself and the structural biases in your systems—biases regarding race, gender, sexual orientation—you can't truly be trauma-informed. Marginalized peoples—excluded, minimized, shamed—are traumatized peoples, because as we've discussed, humans are fundamentally relational creatures. To be excluded or dehumanized in an organization, community, or society you are part of results in prolonged, uncontrollable stress that is sensitizing (see Figure 3). Marginalization is a fundamental trauma.

This is why I believe that a truly trauma-informed system is an anti-racist system. The destructive effects of racial marginalizing are pervasive and severe. In North America, Australia, and New Zealand, for instance, Black, brown, and Indigenous children are more likely to be overdiagnosed and overmedicated in mental health systems; removed from their homes to enter the child welfare system; suspended or expelled from school; and charged at school with truancy and "assault," with the result that they enter the juvenile-justice system in disproportionate ways.

As we've talked about, a child with traumatic experiences will often have difficulty learning—and also be overreactive to the feedback and criticisms that come with struggling in school. This can lead to behavior problems. The behaviors are often misunderstood. So many of the things that people and systems do with good intentions actually cause additional pain for the families and children they're supposed to be serving.

*Oprah*: This is something I want to discuss in a deeper way. During our *60 Minutes* conversation, I realized that so many of the charities and nonprofits out there trying to fix social problems today are really only addressing the surface. They're attempting to build the community scaffolding we know is important, but many are missing the causes—the foundations—of the problems they're trying to solve.

If an after-school program doesn't understand why a child is experiencing chronic health problems or having trouble keeping up in school; if an employment program doesn't figure out why someone is having a hard time with supervisors or always explodes at people— then these programs will not succeed in creating lasting change. Walk us through how some of these issues actually develop and present themselves.

*Dr. Perry*: Let's start with young children. We've talked repeatedly about the important role of early-life relationships in the development of the stress-response systems and the capacity to form future healthy relationships. We know that when children experience distress and trauma—including poverty, homelessness, domestic violence, maltreatment—they will have some disruptions in development. Frequently the result is a "splintering" of the maturation of specific skills, as we talked about in Chapter 6 in relation to neglect. So, a five-year-old child may have only developed the language skills of a typical two-year-old and the self-regulation capabilities of a typical four-year-old. Along with this fragmented development, the child will have an overactive and overly reactive stress response (see Figures 3 and 5).

Now envision this child entering a preschool environment with expectations, transitions, rules, and curricula designed for the typical five-year-old. A developmentally uninformed, trauma-unaware setting will expect this child to "act" typical. But that is impossible for the child. The day will be filled with communication difficulties (due to their language development) and intense frustration (due to their self-regulation capabilities). In this overwhelmingly distressing situation, they will shut down or blow up. Either way, they don't get the full benefit of the social, emotional, or academic learning. They fall further behind. They may be kicked out. More children are expelled from school in pre-K than at any other grade level; children of color, especially boys of color, are expelled at rates three times higher than white children.

This is the start of a toxic mismatch between the child's capabilities and the unrealistic expectations of an education system that is all too often underresourced, developmentally uninformed, and trauma-ignorant. Even if the child "progresses" to the next grade, they are still behind, and this sets them up to fail. Year after year, they fall further and further behind. Their delays in developing skills, together with their trauma-related symptoms, begin to attract mental health labels (see Figure 6). The hypervigilance from their sensitized stress response is labeled ADHD; their predictable efforts to self-regulate—by rocking, chewing gum, doodling, daydreaming, listening to music, tapping their pencil, etc.—are prohibited. They will be labeled, medicated, excluded, punished, perhaps expelled, and then, all too often, arrested. When they try to avoid the constant humiliation of school, they're charged with truancy; when they try to flee and the school staff tries to stop them, a restraint incident results in charges of assault—against the child. This is the school-to-prison pipeline.

*Oprah*: And add to all this the fact that the student most likely has no idea that there's an underlying cause for their struggles. They end up adopting the world's view of them: They are dumb, slow, or lazy. It's a cycle of failure that chips away at their self-esteem until the student becomes so frustrated or ashamed that they give up.

*Dr. Perry*: This is such an important point. A child who is struggling is not going to say, "This poor teacher simply doesn't understand 'state-dependent' functioning and the impact of trauma on my ability to learn. He should be helping me regulate, not conjugate." They say, "I must be dumb."

The other really important point about schools is *how many* children and youth are experiencing learning and behavioral challenges related to trauma. This isn't just a few children; studies show that between 30 and 50 percent of children in public schools have three or more ACEs. And as we've discussed, these adversities have an impact.

Imagine how many children are sitting in school with trauma-related memories that can be activated by innocent cues in the classroom. Remember that what we experience in the present moment is filtered by the lower parts of our brain before getting to the cortex. All incoming sensory information from the present moment is compared to and influenced by the "memories" of previous experiences, and is first processed in the lower, more reactive areas of the brain before reaching the rational, "thinking" areas.

Let's say an older child has grown up with episodic domestic violence; when he was younger he saw his father belittling and hitting his mother. This happened at an important period of brain development, when he was making primary "memories" to make sense of his world. His brain comes to associate attributes of men with threat; a loud, low, masculine voice is connected with fear.

Five years after these associations and memories were made, this young student has a male English teacher who happens to look a little like his abusive father—about the same height, same hair color, deep voice. The boy is not capable of consciously making the connection, but simply sitting in the classroom gives him a feeling of discomfort. This originates in those pre-cortical, lower parts of the brain; it's subconscious. Remember Sam, the boy whose father wore Old Spice? A person is rarely aware when they're activated by an evocative cue.

*Oprah*: And since he's not aware of the association—how what happened to him affects his relationships—he may have a whole history of uncomfortable or sabotaged relationships with the male figures in his life. They may be coaches, teachers, or other men who could be positive role models for him, but he unconsciously avoids or rejects the opportunities.

*Dr. Perry*: It's like when you weren't aware of why you were afraid to be alone at night. You weren't aware of the associations you'd made earlier in your life. Our behaviors begin to shape themselves around the emotional landmines left by previous trauma.

But remember, the brain is always trying to "make sense of the world," so this boy will struggle for an explanation. Maybe he decides he doesn't like English. Or he starts to think that the teacher doesn't like him, that the teacher is a jerk. The teacher has no idea that any of this is happening. So, let's say the student is struggling with a writing assignment. The teacher comes over with the intention of helping; he views his offer of help as a positive thing. As he bends to look at the work, his hand comes to rest on the boy's shoulder. But instead of being calmed, the boy recoils, reacting aggressively before even thinking.

The lower brain immediately says *Danger, danger!* and activates the stress-response system, which immediately shuts down the cortex. So there's no chance for a reasoned, rational response.

Later on, if you talked to the boy and said, "You shouldn't swear at a teacher," he'd say, "I know, it's not a good idea." But in the moment, he truly didn't have access to that ability to reason. The more you learn about trauma and stress response, the easier it is to understand certain behaviors you encounter in a workplace, in a relationship, or at school.

*Oprah*: His brain, triggered by his past association with violence, sends the signal of threat, and he responds with fight or flight: "Get your hands off me!"

*Dr. Perry*: Maybe even "Get your f°ing hands off me!" This aggressive, impulsive lashing out is completely baffling to the teacher. He doesn't understand what is really going on. When he describes the scene to others, he'll say something like, *"For no reason at all, he just came at me."* This is one of the most common descriptions of the behavioral outbursts related to evocative cues: *Out of the blue. Unpredictable.* The behaviors seem unprovoked.

*Oprah*: I just had another *Aha*. So often we use the word *snapped* when we don't know where a burst of anger is coming from or why someone is having a violent reaction. Well, now we know: Something has happened in the moment that triggers one of the brain's trauma memories. And because the lower, non-rational parts of the brain are its first responders, they immediately set off stress responses that then shut off the reasonable part of the brain. And so that "burst" of violence is actually the result of some highly organized processes in the brain. And in this case, the first thing the school is going to say is, *What's wrong with him?*

The teacher, now convinced something *is* wrong with that child, reports him to the principal's office. When what he should be asking is, *What happened to this child?*

*Dr. Perry*: That's right. This child will be viewed as a problem child. And if it continues, he will be sent to see the school counselor, then suspended, then referred to a mental health provider. And if no one in the mental health system understands that his behavioral issues are related to "what happened to him"—related to his trauma—then they will also make a whole set of well-intended but ineffective interventions.

If, on the other hand, this school had the resources and tools to help its teachers understand the prevalence of childhood adversities and the impact of trauma on learning—plus strategies to help create a regulated, safe, and secure classroom—the behavior would have been viewed quite differently. Rather than suspending and labeling the child, the school would try to create a process to connect with and understand him.

*Oprah*: But that only starts if you ask the question: *I wonder what happened to that child?*

*Dr. Perry*: Exactly—if you change how you try to understand behaviors. The good news is that when schools do learn about the effects of trauma and make some simple changes in how they evaluate, support, and teach, they see dramatic improvements in academic achievement and decreases in challenging and disruptive behaviors. If the classroom uses regulatory strategies, the teachers are supported and respected, the needs and strengths of children are identified and addressed, the outcomes are much better.

We work with schools all over the world using our Neurosequential Model in Education (NME), which teaches many of the core concepts you and I have been discussing. NME provides examples of classroom strategies to implement these principles and concepts. The results are very promising. Teachers, administrators, parents, and children all report positive effects, and the outcomes support these views.

Many other groups are introducing "trauma-informed" programs into schools as well. As with the definition of TIC, the elements of these different models and programs vary tremendously. But all of the successful models have one thing in common: They emphasize regulation and connection.

*Oprah*: So helping children regulate is a key "what to do" in a trauma-aware school. Regulate, relate, then reason, yes? Appreciating the sequence of engagement is essential.

*Dr. Perry*: Yes. Unfortunately, our schools are typically not trauma-aware and tend to prohibit many of the regulatory activities we've mentioned: walking, rocking, fiddling with things while listening to a lesson, listening to music with your earbuds while doing homework. "Somatosensory regulation," such as the rhythmic activities we have discussed, actually opens up the cortex and makes the reasoning parts of the brain more accessible for learning.

Schools also tend to minimize powerful healing and resilience-building activities like sports, music, and art. These are often viewed as elective or enrichment activities, when in fact they can be the very bedrock of academic learning, thanks to their regulatory and relational elements. Patterned, repetitive, rhythmic activity makes the overactive and overly reactive core regulatory networks (see Figure 2) get back "in balance." Music falls into this category—both playing and listening. All sports involve doses of it. Dance, too. And, of course, each of these activities also has very important relational elements. You learn when to pass the ball to your teammate; you learn how to move with your dance partner; you synchronize playing your violin with other members of the orchestra. Finally, there are cognitive elements to sports, music, and other arts; they engage, activate, and synchronize activity throughout the brain, from the bottom up and from the top down. These are whole-brain healthy activities.

Now imagine thirty children, sitting in rows in a classroom, passively listening to the teacher lecture. This is not an efficient way to engage the top part of the brain. We learn faster when we're moving and interacting with others. We store new information, and retrieve previously stored information, most efficiently when engaged in some form of somatosensory activation during learning.

*Oprah*: After the student blows up and the school sends them to a mental health service, what happens if that organization has no training or experience with trauma?

*Dr. Perry*: Nothing good. It usually makes the child's situation worse. They are mislabeled and, typically, overmedicated. Our current child mental health systems are underresourced and overwhelmed. It's not uncommon for public menta health clinics to have long waiting lists. Sometimes appointments take place only once a month; sometimes a visit with a psychiatrist lasts only fifteen minutes. The average number of visits before the family simply stops coming is about three. Our mental health systems tend to be crisis-focused.

With that said, there are many places where clinical teams have learned about trauma and are doing really nice work. In the ideal situation, the child will get an assessment that looks at their developmental history—basically, a detailed evaluation of "what happened to you?" A good assessment will also determine the child's needs and strengths. Based upon these, the team can create an individual treatment approach that will take advantage of the child's strengths and target the areas of need with appropriate enrichment, educational, or therapeutic activities.

These teams know that any "one size fits all" solution does not work. Think about how absurd it would be if everyone who had chest pain and a cough got the exact same antibiotic. That is what happens in many clinics that specialize in a specific "technique." At a clinic that has learned that trauma-focused cognitive behavioral therapy (TF-CBT) is an evidence-based intervention for trauma, everyone with trauma may get this intervention. But while it is helpful for some, it isn't for all.

A truly trauma-aware clinical team has a lot of "tools" to use: occupational therapy, physical therapy, speech and language supports, liaisons with the school, good psychoeducation with the family and child, plus access to a range of therapeutic techniques such as TF-CBT, Eye Movement Desensitization and Reprocessing (EMDR), somatosensory interventions, animal-assisted therapies, and many more. Despite being a young field, traumatology does have preliminary evidence of the effectiveness of many of these techniques when used at the *right time* in the treatment process.

What that means is that an effective therapeutic approach has to follow the *sequence of engagement;* problems with regulating have to be addressed before you can get results with relational or cognitive therapies. This is why I developed the Neurosequential Model of Therapeutics (NMT) that I wrote about in my first book with Maia Szalavitz, *The Boy Who Was Raised as a Dog.*

For me, one of the most important aspects of healing is recognizing that it can involve multiple therapeutic techniques and approaches. What we know is that the key ingredient of effective healing involves using your healthy relationships to revisit and rework the traumatic experience. If you have a therapist and form a safe and stable connection, the therapist becomes a critical part of what I call your "therapeutic web." But remember that therapeutic moments can be brief and ideally are spread throughout your whole week—it's not just about one hour a week with the therapist. This process creates opportunities to activate trauma memories, including the stress-response systems, in a moderate, predictable, and controllable way. In turn, this will take the sensitized systems and, over time, make them more "neurotypical" (see Figures 3 and 5).

*Oprah*: What if you don't have the resources to get a therapist?

*Dr. Perry*: Great question. Most people who experience adversity and trauma do *not* have access to therapy, let alone a clinical team like I just described. But what we're learning is that having access to a number of invested, caring people is actually a better predictor of good outcomes following trauma than having access to a therapist. The therapeutic web is the collection of positive relational-based opportunities you have throughout your day. A therapist can be an important part of healing, but isn't required. This isn't to suggest that therapy isn't helpful, but therapy without "connectedness" is not very effective. Ideally, a child can have connectedness to family, community, and culture, along with a trauma-aware clinical team and its range of tools.

And again, if you look at Indigenous and traditional healing practices, they do a remarkable job of creating a total mind-body experience that influences multiple brain systems. Remember, trauma "memories" span multiple brain areas. So these traditional practices will have cognitive, relational-based, and sensory elements. You retell the story; create images of the battle, hunt, death; hold each other; massage; dance; sing. You reconnect to loved ones—to community. You celebrate, eat, and share. Aboriginal healing practices are repetitive, rhythmic, relevant, relational, respectful, and rewarding—experiences known to be effective in altering neural systems involved in the stress response. The practices emerged because they worked. People felt better and functioned better, and the core elements of the healing process were reinforced and passed on. Cultures separated by time and space converged on the same principles for healing.

*Oprah*: When you think about it, that really is remarkable.

*Dr. Perry*: It is. Our ancestors recognized the importance of connectedness and the toxicity of exclusion. The history of the "civilized" world, on the other hand, is filled with policies and practices that favored disconnection and marginalization—that destroyed family, community, and culture. Colonization, slavery, the U.S. reservation system, Canada's Residential Schools, Australia's Stolen Generation—these were so destructive across so many generations because they intentionally destroyed the family and cultural bonds that keep a people connected. They created disconnected, traumatized individuals in inescapable, painful situations—situations that, as we've discussed, make people dissociate in order to adapt and survive. And even though the dissociation is adaptive, it results in more passivity and compliance, making traumatized peoples easier to dehumanize and exploit.

While less obvious to some, I believe that our existing child-welfare, educational, mental health, and juvenile-justice systems often do the same thing. They fragment families, undermine community, and engage in marginalizing, shaming, and punitive practices.

*Oprah*: You spoke so movingly about systemic racism, dismantled power, and trauma when you joined me in South Africa once to visit my school. We'd built the Oprah Winfrey Leadership Academy for Girls in 2007, thirteen years after the formal end of apartheid and the creation of a democratic South African government. When you visited, we were struggling to create a healthy sense of community among the faculty.

The Black teachers felt that the white teachers expressed a level of superiority even though they were accepting of them. You provided so much clarity when you explained what might be going on between the two groups using the lens of brain development and its connection to implicit bias and racism. Can you do that here?

*Dr. Perry*: Of course. We have talked about how an infant's brain takes in sensory information to make sense of their world and build associations. And we've talked about how we're deeply relational creatures whose developing brains—starting with the lowest areas—begin to make "memories" of the smells, sounds, and images of "our people."

These memories exist on a very deep, pre-cortical, unconscious level: the way your people talk, the way they dress, the color of their skin.

Now remember that your brain is always monitoring your world—both inside and outside—to ensure your survival. And when the brain encounters any unfamiliar experience, its default move is to activate the stress response. Better to be safe than sorry—better to assume that novelty can be a potential threat.

Now add to this the fact that the major predator of humans has always been other humans. Our stress response has evolved to be relationally sensitive, such that when we're with people who have attributes similar to our childhood "clan," we feel safe. But when we encounter people with attributes that are different from "our people," the brain's default is to activate the stress response. When that happens, we feel dysregulated, even threatened.

*Oprah*: This is why, if you have a new baby and everyone wants to see the baby and is passing the baby around, sometimes the baby will start crying. Their brain is reacting to the unfamiliar.

*Dr. Perry*: Absolutely. To the infant, all these people are different, new, and overwhelming. That activates a stress response.

But adult brains also activate the stress response in reaction to people who are different from their original "clan." Now, most of the time this activation is mild, creating a wariness, caution. But if someone has a sensitized stress response or the attributes of the new person are very different from your clan, a more dramatic stress activation can take place. And when that happens, we regress. We lose access to the higher part of our brain, the part that stores our values and beliefs. Our thinking and behavior start to be driven by more primitive, reactive parts of our brain.

Let me give an example. I once met a woman whose daughter joined the Peace Corps and was going from village to village in a very rural area of Africa giving children immunizations. She was from Minnesota and very Scandinavian-looking: tall, blonde, pale white skin.

*Oprah*: And she'd go into villages where people had literally never seen a white person.

*Dr. Perry*: Yes. So here is this very positive, big-hearted young woman who loves children and feels like she's making the world a better place, enthusiastically going into rural villages to combat disease. But when she'd walk into a village, the young children would take one look at her and scream. They thought she was a ghost. Some of them would start crying, some would run away. This was hard for the young woman to get used to. And it wasn't until her mother told her about some of our work that she finally understood that these children were reacting to the "unknown" and not to her personally. Their brains had not created any positive associations to "whiteness," so encountering her was very unexpected and stress-activating.

But that's only the initial response. Over time, the young woman is loving to them, nurtures them, takes care of them. She helps feed them, and regulates them when they're scared. So the children learn that this white person who's giving them love and nurturing and support is safe and good. And that learning gets "locked" into their brain to the point that if they have an encounter years later with another white person, their default will be to categorize the new white person as positive.

*Oprah*: Even if the new white person is not so nice, it won't necessarily undo the original template of the nice white lady from Minnesota, because that template was built more deeply into their brain at a young age.

*Dr. Perry*: That's right. The first time you encounter someone with characteristics—such as skin color—that are unlike "your people," you begin to create new associations to help you make sense of your world because your world now includes a new person. Your brain will sort, compare, and categorize this person. In the beginning, it will use your existing defaults—this is a person with male attributes, this is a person older than I am, this is a person who is a teacher. But the more times you're with this person, the more chances you have to build new, more nuanced associations. You get to know the facets and complexities of the person, and not simply their "categories."

At the same time, though, the brain is always using "shortcuts." And these shortcuts are not always accurate; they make us vulnerable to stereotypes and "isms"—generalizing attributes of people based upon the broad categories they fall into. And the most powerful categories in our brain come from our first experiences, usually in early life. This contributes to our tendencies for bias.

A while back, when I was working with a young Black child, I asked him if he had ever met a white man.

"One," he said.

It turned out that the first white person this boy really saw up close—not on television—was a police officer who pulled his dad over, aimed his gun at his dad, made his dad get out of the car, yelled at his dad, handcuffed him, and then threw his dad into the squad car. The boy was left sitting in the car, terrified, until a social worker showed up and took him away. They didn't even let his mother see him until she had "proven" who she was. You can imagine that the boy's internal representation of white people was very different from the village children's after they were nurtured by the white Peace Corps volunteer.

Now this same child—the one who watched his father being violently arrested—later comes to see me, a white doctor who is trying to help him. Our relationship doesn't start from a neutral place. He feels fearful, distrusting of me—in part because I'm new to him, in part because I'm white. It takes weeks and weeks of gentle, patient, positive work before he can view me as neutral. We did end up connecting in good ways, but I was viewed as an exception. His original negative experiences with whiteness, reinforced by many related experiences of overt and implicit racism at school and in the community, stayed with him. The earliest relational experiences are the most powerful and enduring.

Because of the sequential processing of experience, this boy will always process "whiteness" in the lower part of his brain first. When he encounters a new white man, his original—and therefore default—association of white men and threat will cause a stress activation that can influence how he feels, thinks, and behaves. It's like an evocative cue. The boy's brain has already activated his fear response by the time any other information about the new white man can get to his cortex. In his cortex, he does have some autobiographical memory from seeing me, some stored information that *"Dr. Perry is white, but he was okay."* But in the moment, with an activated fear response, he cannot efficiently access that information. He will look at this new white man and feel, *"But this isn't Dr. Perry."* Our first experiences create the filters through which all new experiences must pass.

In the case of South Africa, there are many, many cultures in one country. And for generations, the white community brutally oppressed people of color. The Black teachers at OWLAG had grown up in a world where active resistance to white power and the country's racist policies, practices, and laws could lead to death. Associations related to whiteness were often fear-inducing. Many Black people developed an adaptive strategy and style that was fundamentally dissociative. Avoid conflict; when confronted, comply. Adaptive capabilities like these are deeply ingrained.

*Oprah*: And so many of the teachers in the school may have unconsciously been holding on to those old ways of thinking and behaving.

*Dr. Perry*: Exactly. In 1994, when the oppressive practices of apartheid ended, people's brains didn't immediately change. White people were still associated with dominance and marginalization. Even though things had theoretically changed, when people who were raised in apartheid interacted with each other, there was an unconscious reestablishing of power differentials, and an eliciting of old patterns of adaptation. The white teachers felt comfortable speaking up and "leading"; the Black teachers sat back, avoided conflict, and complied with suggestions they didn't necessarily support. This led to big problems at the school. And yet when I talked to the white teachers, they would sincerely say that racism was not playing a role in the issues at the school.

One of the hardest things to grasp about implicit bias and racism is that your beliefs and values do not always drive your behavior. These beliefs and values are stored in the highest, most complex part of your brain—the cortex. But other parts of your brain can make associations—distorted, inaccurate, racist associations. The same person can have very sincere anti-racist beliefs but still have implicit biases that result in racist comments or actions. Understanding sequential processing in the brain is essential to grasping this, as is appreciating the power of developmental experiences to load the lower parts of our brain with all kinds of associations that create our worldview.

*Oprah*: We hear so many white people say, "Nobody ever used the N-word in my house." But it's not just a matter of language. It's how you see your parents treat people who are not like you. It's how you see them in their interactions with other people. It's what is said about them. It's the emotional tone that comes through in your household about people who are "other." That is what you're taking in from the time you're born, so it shapes how you see people who aren't like you. Whether somebody used the N-word or didn't use the N-word isn't the point. There are a lot more influences at work.

*Dr. Perry*: Many more. When you're young and you're forming your primary associations about how the world works, your major influences come from your parents. And not really what they say, but how they act. You're also influenced by the other children and adults around you. If you're a white child who spends no time with children of color, you don't have any personal experiences to help build those important relational associations.

We're also profoundly influenced by the media. From infancy, the media images we see shape our understanding of the world. For many white people, their only experience or perception of people of color is through the media. When I was growing up, the media was permeated with negative stereotypes about Black people.

*Oprah*: I know lots of white people who, until they met me, had never known a Black person. And there was a time when some white people actually had Black people working for them so they could say they knew one. But as you say, for many white people, their only association with Black people was what they saw on the news or in the movies.

*Dr. Perry*: When I was young, Black men and Black youth in movies or on TV were much more likely to be portrayed in a negative way—as a criminal, for example. They weren't the detectives, superheroes, scientists. This distortion has an incredibly powerful impact on the way your brain organizes. It contributes to the negative associations white people create about people of color; it is a big part of creating implicit bias.

We all create our own version of the world that has distortions. As I said, the brain's shortcuts in processing information make us vulnerable to bias. Everybody has some form of implicit bias—some distortion of the world—that's based on how and where they grew up. Imagine the odds of having every single culture and every single religion and every single ethnicity become part of your "safe and familiar" catalog—let alone being exposed to all that in the first few years of life. And so we need to acknowledge that we all carry some of these things around.

*Oprah*: In Isabel Wilkerson's book *Caste,* she quotes a study from a criminal-justice reform organization called the Sentencing Project. They found that crimes involving a Black suspect and a white victim make up only 10 percent of all crimes—but they account for 42 percent of what's reported on television. When you're watching the news and almost half of what you see is Black people committing crimes against white people, that's going to influence the way you think when you see a Black person.

*Dr. Perry*: Let's take a moment to think of how that implicit bias plays a role in an interaction between an inexperienced white cop in a confrontation with a Black teenager late at night. It's a matter of state-dependent functioning. Under threat, the reasoning part of the brain starts to shut down, and the more reactive, emotional parts of the brain take over. Say you're the white cop and you feel threatened and you have a gun. If the lower, more reactive parts of your brain start to dominate your cognitions and behaviors when you feel under threat, and your brain has a whole catalog of Black men as threatening criminals, you are much more likely to engage in fear-based behavior—yelling, escalating, pulling a trigger—with a Black teen than with a white teen. Your brain isn't filled with a catalog of threatening white teens.

Talk about a system that needs trauma training. Law enforcement should be at the top of the list. Training about trauma, the brain, stress, and distress is essential if you are going to be a first responder—especially a police officer. Anyone given the responsibility of carrying a gun in service of society should have extensive training in these things.

*Oprah*: But there is a difference between implicit bias and racism. Where do you see that line?

*Dr. Perry*: Implicit bias suggests that the bias is present but not "plainly expressed"—sometimes even unintentionally expressed. Racism, on the other hand, is an actual overt set of beliefs about the superiority of one race over others. In the U.S., racism is the marginalization and oppression of people of color by systems created by white men to privilege white people. You could say that racism is embedded in the top, "rational" part of your brain, whereas implicit bias involves the distorting "filters" created in lower parts of the brain. When a child or youth is exposed to overt racist beliefs, possibly in their home or peer groups, those beliefs can become "embedded" in the filters. The result can be a deeply ingrained set of feelings and beliefs that cut across multiple regions of the brain.

*Oprah*: Change, however, is possible. I think it's important to bring up a conversation I had in 2018 that confirmed my belief that through compassion, there is hope for even the most racist individual to evolve.

I spoke with a man named Anthony Ray Hinton, who'd spent thirty years on death row in Alabama for a crime he didn't commit. The prison setup was extremely isolating—just him alone in his cell, unable to see any of the other inmates on the row with him. No one ever really talked to each other, but at night you could hear crying and moaning—men in pain.

One night, Anthony heard someone crying, and something inside him shifted. He called out: *"What's wrong?"* And the man told him that his mother had died.

Now, Anthony was extremely close to his own mother, and in that moment, he empathized. And that one question, that act of compassion, opened the door for all the men. They began talking to each other regularly, sharing stories, giving each other support. Anthony became particularly friendly with a man named Henry. And he eventually learned that his friend Henry was Henry Hays, a member of the KKK who'd been imprisoned for hanging a young Black boy. But instead of cutting him off and ending the friendship, Anthony formed a bond with him on death row, and they remained close friends.

*Dr. Perry*: I would bet that by doing that, Anthony was able to also change Henry.

*Oprah*: So much so that on the night Henry was electrocuted, his last words were that all of his life, he'd gotten it wrong. His parents had taught him wrong, that Black people were the enemy. And he'd had to come to death row to learn what love was.

*Dr. Perry*: Wow. That's incredibly powerful. And a perfect example of how even the most hateful racist belief system can be changed.

Remember that the cortex is the most malleable, the most changeable part of the brain. Beliefs and values can change.

*Oprah*: Implicit bias is trickier to change, right?

*Dr. Perry*: Implicit bias is much more difficult. You may truly believe that racism is bad, that all people are equal. But those beliefs are in the intellectual part of your brain, and your implicit biases, which are in the lower part of your brain, will still play out every day—in the way you interact with others, the jokes you laugh at, the things you say.

It is interesting to watch how this relates to the Black Lives Matter movement. In the wake of the murder of George Floyd, so many conversations have been sparked about structural racism, implicit bias, and white privilege. This has illuminated so much misunderstanding and resulted in so much expressed pain. And, of course, so much defensiveness. "I've never been racist." "I don't have a racist bone in my body." Well, the issue isn't your bones. It's your brain. All of us have deeply ingrained biases, and lurking among these are racist associations.

The challenge of addressing implicit bias is first recognizing that you have it. Reflect on when your biases have been expressed. Anticipate when and where you may be likely to express your bias. Be courageous enough to spend time with people who are different from you and who may challenge your biases. It can be uncomfortable. But remember: Moderate, predictable, controllable stress can build resilience. Create new associations; have new experiences. Ideally, you go out into the community and spend time with people who are different than you are. You need to create real, meaningful relationships so that you get to know individuals based on their unique qualities, not based on categories.

*Oprah*: That's what really changes both implicit bias and racism.

*Dr. Perry*: Exactly. And this is why you can't be in a corporation and address these issues by simply having everyone go to an anti-racism course or cultural-sensitivity training. You don't get trained in cultural sensitivity—you go spend time immersed in the culture, spend time with other people. Anthony Bourdain was a great example of this. He encouraged people to experience other cultures by spending time with the cooks, preparing the meals, eating the food, celebrating cultural events with the people who celebrate them. You can't become culturally sensitive from a three-hour seminar.

*Oprah*: Does that mean that we shouldn't have cultural-sensitivity training?

*Dr. Perry:* No, it means that cultural-sensitivity training, which may help get at the intellectual elements of learning, needs to be coupled with real experiences and real relationships. That is what will help change you. It's hard for many people to do, and it certainly doesn't fix the whole system, but it's a start.

The long-term solution is to minimize the development of implicit bias. We have to think about ways to raise our children with more opportunities to be exposed to the magnificence of human diversity earlier in their lives. And we have to change the inherently biased elements of so many of our systems.

*Oprah:* Do you think that trauma is causing humanity to move backward?

*Dr. Perry:* As we discussed earlier, human beings have always lived with a lot of trauma. So despite all of the challenges we've been talking about, I'm optimistic. I think the "humanity" of our species ebbs and flows; there have been times of tremendous humanity and times of terrible inhumanity. But if you look at the history of human-kind, all the major indicators related to health and welfare, social justice, creativity, and productivity are trending up right now.

This isn't to say that now isn't an incredibly hard time in the United States. There is a lot of polarization; there are a lot of people using fear to shape public opinion. Angry, polarized groups don't listen well, but they are communicating fear and pain and hunger for change.

I'm hopeful that by teaching about trauma and the power of con-nectedness, things will improve. We could invest in building neigh-borhoods, building trauma-informed services, supporting artists, rebuilding the infrastructure, building spaces where people would create community. We could have a quantum leap in humanity. We could. We can. But first we need to understand the pervasive and complex effects of trauma. We have so much unexpressed potential.

# CHAPTER 9

# RELATIONAL HUNGER IN THE MODERN WORLD

*The Māori elder walked us to a gate at the bottom of a gentle sloping hill. At the top of the hill was a beautiful rectangular building with amazing carvings on its pillars and beams. The gate led into the* marae, *an enclosed area that is the center of Māori community life. The building was the community meeting house, or* wharenui. *Several dozen members of the Māori community lined the path up to the meeting house. One of the elders approached us holding a club and loudly speaking Māori, then placed a frond on the ground in front of me. An elder woman started to sing. Others joined in; our welcoming ceremony, the* pōwhiri, *had started.*

*Twenty-five years ago, Dr. Robin Fancourt, a pioneer of pediatrics in New Zealand, asked me to come visit and teach about my work on developmental trauma and the brain. In return, I had asked if she could help arrange time with some Māori healers. I had been trying to understand more about the healing practices of Indigenous peoples. Trauma has always been part of the human journey, and our ancestors knew trauma well. I'd spent some time listening to and learning from elders and healers from First Nations, Métis, and Native American communities. I'd seen common elements of healing practices—most prominently, the use of rhythm and an emphasis on harmony with nature. I knew, though, that there was much more to understand.*

*For the next two days I was going to learn about trauma and healing through the lens of a Māori community. My first lesson was about education. The elders didn't have me sit and read or give me a "presentation" about traditional healing. They immersed me in community for two days. In their wisdom, they were gifting me a learning opportunity, an experience. What I could discover was profound, but what I would discover was on me. Would I let myself be open enough to truly learn—or would I simply filter the experience through my Western medicine lens and regard it as a quaint anthropological footnote?*

*For the rest of the first day and night, the community came together on the marae. We gathered in the meetinghouse, sat on the floor. Many talked with me about traditional ways. Very quickly it was clear that they made no conceptual separation of problems or solutions into categories like education, mental health, juvenile justice, or child welfare. There was a wholeness to their ways of thinking and being. This was remarkably similar to the "worldview" that Cree and Métis elders had shared with me. There was also a true appreciation of our journey to this moment, an awareness that in order to best understand the here and now, we need to know where we come from and "what happened" to us and our ancestors.*

*When someone spoke to the group, they went to a corner where everyone could see them and they could see everyone. The speaker introduced themselves by tracing their family lineages, frequently noting an ancestor's special attribute; this explicit tracing of ancestral heritage brought a continuous appreciation of cross-generational connections. Then they would speak, often using storytelling to make a key point.*

*Throughout the two days, there were communal meals. These were a mix of ceremony, conversation, games, storytelling—all with lots of laughing and hugging. It had the feeling of a family reunion. The warmth and strength of the community were palpable. At night we all slept in the* wharenui, *together, as a community.*

*On both days, I had the honor of being guided onto the land and walking the forest and beach with two of the elder healers. At times they would stop, walk off the path to a plant, and break off a leaf or some bark, or dig for a root. They would have me smell and taste, telling me about the potential uses. "Make a paste with seawater." "This helps with pain."*

*The elders were very patient with my curiosity, and gently amused at my Western medical-model formulations of "disease" when I asked how they handled depression, sleep problems, drug abuse, and trauma. They kept trying to help me understand that these problems were all basically the "same thing." The problems were all* interconnected. *In Western psychiatry we like to separate them, but that misses the true essence of the problem. We are chasing symptoms, not healing people.*

*For my Māori hosts, pain, distress, and dysfunction would arise from some form of fragmentation, disconnection, dyssynchrony. We talked extensively about these issues. The Māori people, like all colonized peoples of the world, have been impacted greatly by historical trauma. The transgenerational fallout of colonization, cultural genocide, and racism has been devastating. Rates of unemployment, poverty, alcoholism, domestic violence, mental health, and physical health problems are much higher among the Māori than in the general population of New Zealand (which is 85 percent white). Similar overrepresentation of Indigenous people and people of color in special-education, mental health, juvenile-justice, and criminal-justice systems is seen in Australia with Aboriginal and Torres Strait peoples, Canada with First Nations, and the United States with Black, Latinx, and Native American populations. The Māori concept of "disease" explained these differences better than my medical model did; colonization intentionally fragments families, community cohesion, and cultures, and that disconnection is at the heart of trauma.*

*A core element of all of the traditional healing practices was something the Māori called* whanaungatanga. *The word refers to reciprocal relationships, kinship, and a sense of family connection. From shared experiences and challenges, a sense of connectedness and belonging emerges. Many of the healing practices and rituals involve "reconnection"—explicit articulation of the origins of connection. This involves sharing experiences such as a hunt or raid and then symbolically and literally reconnecting to family, community, and the natural world.*

*The elders were always clear that they were not rejecting advances in genetics, immunology, or physiology, and they partnered closely with the Western-trained physicians working in their community.*

*But they felt that a view of health that granulated the complexity of a person into component parts—treated by the bone doctor, eye doctor, brain doctor, and so on—was simply missing the core elements of health. If connectedness—whanaungatanga— wasn't addressed, the potential effectiveness of Western interventions was blunted.*

*As my visit was coming to an end, I stood next to the elder on a bluff overlooking the ocean. Wind was blowing off from the water; waves were crashing against the rocks. The effect was loud, overpowering, and rhythmic. I thanked the elder for spending so much time with me; she turned to me and smiled. She put her palm over my heart and said, "We are healers." At the time, fueled by my Western-physician ego, I thought she meant that she and I were healers. Now I understand that she was trying to tell me, once again, that the collective "we" of a community heals. We are all healers.*

*When I returned from New Zealand, I was determined to better understand the "relational health" of the children I worked with. I was curious to see if we could find evidence of the correlations between health and connectedness. The first step was recognizing that I hadn't really been asking about some of the most important aspects of the children's lives. How did they spend their time—all day? Who were their friends, their "people"? Where did they feel safe? And what had happened along the way that resulted in their being sent to a psychiatrist? I had been too focused on "what was wrong" with them—what problems, symptoms, failures in school we needed to address. Our standard assessments measured the nature and severity of their symptoms. We didn't measure the nature and quality of their relationships. Our approach to treatment wasn't getting to the heart of healing—whanaungatanga.*

*Timothy, a ten-year-old boy, was one of the first patients I talked with after coming back from New Zealand. We had been seeing him in our clinic for about nine months; he'd been referred by a local pediatrician after being involved in several angry outbursts and aggressive behavior with a classmate. He had been given a diagnosis of ADHD and oppositional defiant disorder (ODD); the medications prescribed to "treat" his "disorders" had not improved his symptoms, hence the referral to our clinic.*

*When I looked back at his records, I saw many clues to his current problems. Starting at age three, Timothy had been physically abused by his mother's live-in partner. They lived with this violence and abuse for about three years, until his mother left the abusive partner—at which point they were immediately plunged into poverty. His mom struggled to find a decent job. Over the next three years, they moved to three different cities—resulting in three new schools for Timothy, three new neighborhoods and sets of neighbors. Finally, after they moved to Texas, his mom got steady work. Slowly they started to regain some economic and social stability. But their experiences had taken a serious toll on both of them.*

*The mother was worn out and worn down, depressed but functioning, barely. Timothy had classic trauma-related symptoms: hypervigilance mislabeled as ADHD, sleep issues, exhaustion from the sleep issues and his continuously overactive stress response. And then there was the social immaturity. Despite being ten years old, Timothy had grown up with few opportunities for social "practice." The combination of always being the new kid and having a trauma-related inefficiency in learning led to a significant delay in his socio-emotional development. He was like a five-year-old in a ten-year-old social world. He was ignored or teased. He was excluded. He felt most regulated when he was alone or with his mom. He wanted to fit in with other people, but he didn't have the skills. When they first moved to Texas, he'd made friends with a six-year-old on his block, but this boy's parents were uncomfortable with the age difference and discouraged, then forbade, any significant play together.*

*At the clinic, Timothy and I sat at a table together, in parallel, drawing and coloring.*

*"You know, I realized that I never asked you about your friends,"
I ventured.*

*He kept coloring, didn't say a word. Almost as if he hadn't heard
me, but I knew he was using an avoidant response.*

*"Who is your best friend?"*

*Without hesitation he said, "Raymond is my best friend."*

*"I don't remember you talking about Raymond."*

*"He is really nice. We went swimming together. And caught some
frogs. He likes Ninja Turtles like me." Though he was usually somewhat withdrawn and sad-looking, Timothy was animated and enthusiastic now.*

*"Are you guys in the same class?"*

*He stopped, seemed to be thinking. "I don't know. I didn't ask."*

*I was confused. "Does he go to your school?"*

*"No. He lives in Kansas."*

*"Ah. How often do you guys get together?"*

*"Just last summer. Maybe I'll see him next summer when we go
camping again," he said wistfully, returning to his sad baseline.*

*I felt sad as well. Here was a child telling me his best friend was
someone he'd met once at a campground and played with for a few
days. This boy had no friends, really. His extended family lived in
a different city, he wasn't part of a community of faith, he was a
single child, and he was marginalized within the school because of
his immature and impulsive behaviors. He was viewed as an "odd"
child. His mother worked so hard, struggling all alone to care for
him. When I saw her, she always looked sad herself.*

*The contrast between their world and the Māori community was
striking. The Māori had such rich relational density and developmental diversity—babies, children, youth, adults, and elderly all in the
same space, moving, singing, talking, eating, laughing. I imagined
Timothy running around the marae with other children, episodically
engaging with aunties, uncles, and grandparents. Or camping again*

*and chasing frogs with his friend Raymond. It made me smile. Then, more realistically, I pictured him searching the school cafeteria for a safe place to sit alone at lunch; walking home from school to an empty apartment; waiting for his tired, loving mother to come home; filling the time with video games and TV.*

*Trauma had impacted both Timothy and his mother. They were both experiencing poverty of relationships. They had no therapeutic web of positive relationships, the relationships needed for healing. Timothy and his mother needed connection—they needed* whanaungatanga.

*Over the next weeks, we met with Timothy and his mother several times and changed our treatment approach. First, we enrolled the mother in our clinic. As surprising as it sounds, few clinics for children also serve adults. Considering the frequency of transgenerational and intra-family trauma, this is a powerful example of the destructive fragmentation of our "siloed" systems. We found Timothy an in-school mentor, signed him up for an after-school program with the Boys & Girls Club in his neighborhood, and stopped all his medications. We encouraged his mom to check out a local church's group for single parents; she had grown up as a Presbyterian but hadn't really found a "church home" in Texas. We met with several of Timothy's teachers as part of an individual educational plan (IEP). After learning what lay beneath his behaviors, the teachers were much more understanding, and one took a special interest in him. Timothy had been invisible, and the teachers were all overextended. But now he was "seen" by more people at school.*

*Six months later, Timothy was thriving. He had no more behavior problems at school, and he'd made up a full year of academic content. He had a new best friend, someone he played with every week. He was active in school, after school, and in his new community of faith. His mom was also doing better. She found the single-parent group very helpful and was forming new friendships. She had been heartbroken by Timothy's struggles, so his progress was a tonic for her. And the natural contagion of a happier parent only fed his progress. Positive reciprocal relationships and a new sense of belonging helped heal this small family. It was just the beginning of my exploration of the power of connectedness.*

—Dr. Perry

*Oprah*: You have said that our world is relationally impoverished. We live in environments where we see fewer people, and even when we do see people and engage in conversation, we're not really listening to each other or being fully present. And this disconnection is making us more vulnerable.

*Dr. Perry*: I think that's true. Even though we live in an amazing country filled with good people, I believe that collectively we're less resilient. Our ability as a people to tolerate stressors is diminishing because our connectedness is diminishing.

This relational poverty means less buffering capacity when we do experience stress. We are becoming more "sensitized" to anything that feels potentially threatening, such as a person with a different political opinion. Many people are overly reactive to relatively minor challenges. And when we're overly sensitive as a result of state-dependent functioning, we quickly shift to a less rational, more emotional style of thinking and acting. We're losing the ability to calmly consider someone else's opinion, reflect, and attempt to see things from their point of view.

*Oprah*: I see that all the time. Someone makes one mistake, or something they said a long time ago resurfaces, and "cancel culture" takes over. No one wants to listen to each other.

*Dr. Perry*: The irony is that all human communication is characterized by moments of miscommunication and getting out of sync, but then repairing things. As my good friend Ed Tronick, a pioneer in developmental psychology, teaches us, interpersonal rupture and repair is good for building resilience. These ruptures are perfect doses of moderate, controllable stress.

Conversation, for example, promotes resilience; discussions and arguments over family dinners and mildly heated conversations with friends are—as long as there is repair—resilience-building and empathy-growing experiences. We shouldn't be walking away from a conversation in a rage; we should regulate ourselves. Repair the ruptures. Reconnect and grow. When you walk away, everybody loses. We all need to get better at listening, regulating, reflecting. This requires the capacity to forgive, to be patient. Mature human interactions involve efforts to understand people who are different from you. But if we don't have family meals, don't go out with friends for long, in-person conversations, and communicate only via text or Twitter, then we can't create that positive, healthy back-and-forth pattern of human connection.

*Oprah*: Pleasant, positive moments are wonderful, of course. But what you're saying is that true growth comes from tougher moments, more difficult conversations. And we need to approach these moments with an awareness of "What happened to you?"

*Dr. Perry*: Empathy is the ability to put yourself in somebody else's shoes—both in an emotional sense, to feel a bit of what they may feel, but also in a cognitive sense, to see the situation from their perspective. If you approach an interaction from an empathic stance, you're much less likely to have a negative perspective on whatever is going on. And hopefully that will allow you to get to know the person better—even if it's someone you already know. Hopefully you get to know more of their story, and this in turn lets you be a bit more regulated in the way you interact with them.

When somebody is being rude, our typical response is to get caught up in the contagion of their emotions—we get dysregulated and then we mirror their rude behaviors. But if you can approach the interaction from a regulated, empathic stance, your response changes.

*Oprah*: And that changes everything. You've also said that the human brain is really not designed for the modern world. Let's talk about that.

*Dr. Perry*: Well, human beings have been human beings—in this genetic form—for about 250,000 years. And for 99.9 percent of that time, we lived in hunter-gatherer bands of relatively small multifamily groups. So our brain is "suited" for the social attributes and complexities of these smaller groups. Through almost the entirety of our existence as humans, our social "network" was small—we only "knew" sixty to one hundred people. We may have had some connection to other bands with similar kinship ties and some common cultural elements, but mostly our "world" was small and embedded in the natural world. We had more developmental diversity—adults, youth, and children mixing in the same spaces throughout the day. There was more physical proximity, more touch, more connectedness.

The daily rhythms, colors, light, and sounds of the natural world are what our sensory systems evolved to monitor, as well as the verbal and even more so nonverbal cues of our relatively small but complex social groups—our clans and tribes.

But today we live very differently than we did thousands of years ago. We have invented our modern world. And whenever this world and its inventions start to stretch us away from our genetic capabilities and preferences, we run into problems.

Our current challenge is that the rate of invention is now exceeding the rate at which we can problem-*solve*. In the last two thousand years, the rate of change in our world—in our demographics, technology, transportation, etc.—has exploded. As the writer and biochemist Isaac Asimov said, "The saddest aspect of life right now is that science gathers knowledge faster than society gathers wisdom."

Part of the challenge of inventing ourselves away from the natural world and our "social" preferences is that doing so stresses the neural systems involved in monitoring the world. Our stress-response systems are drained by constantly monitoring the sensory cacophony of the modern world: street sounds, traffic, airplanes, radios, TVs, the hum of refrigerators, the hiss of computer fans. Living in an urban environment taxes these systems even more: Every time you see someone new on the street, your brain asks, *Safe and familiar? Friend or foe? Trustworthy or not?*—over and over and over again. You scan the attributes of each person and compare them to your "internal catalog" of "safe and familiar." This constant monitoring of the social environment can consume a significant portion of our bandwidth.

At the same time, we're in rebellion against nature. We use artificial light to stay awake at night. The foods we eat are extremely processed—profoundly different from the foods that our bodies evolved to digest. All of this stresses our body, especially the brain.

And the stress is far worse if you have to also worry about housing, food, or employment. The unpredictability and insecurities of poverty drain the stress-response system's bandwidth in ways that make "opportunities" to escape poverty extremely difficult to take advantage of.

*Oprah*: We've talked about how poverty can induce trauma. But as you're pointing out, it's not just economic poverty that we have to worry about. Isolation and loneliness are an epidemic.

*Dr. Perry*: Yes, I'm very concerned about poverty of relationships in modern society. In our work, we find that the best predictor of your current mental health is your current "relational health," or connectedness. This connectedness is fueled by two things: the basic capabilities you've developed to form and maintain relationships, and the relational "opportunities" you have in your family, neighborhood, school, and so forth.

Simply put, modern life provides fewer opportunities for relational interactions. In a multifamily, multigenerational environment, the continuous social interactions provide a rich source of regulation, reward, and learning. And that's how we used to live. In 1790, 63 percent of our nation's households had five or more people; only

10 percent had two or fewer. Today those numbers have basically flipped: In 2006, only 8 percent of households had five or more people; 60 percent had two or fewer. In a recent survey of selected urban communities in the U.S., Europe, and Japan, up to 60 percent of all households were just one person.

Add to this the impact of screen time. At home, at work, at school, we spend hours and hours in front of a screen—on average, over 11 hours a day. We are having far fewer family meals; our conversational skills are fading. The art of storytelling and the capacity to listen are on the decline. The result is a more self-absorbed, more anxious, more depressed—and less resilient—population.

*Oprah*: Do you think all of this adds up to less empathy?

*Dr. Perry*: Well, the capacity to demonstrate empathy is a function of key neural networks in the brain, and these networks are organized on a use-dependent basis. In other words, just as language fluency requires exposure to lots of conversation and verbal stimulation, "empathic fluency" requires sufficient repetition with caring relational interactions. And our modern world is not providing these opportunities for our children.

In extreme situations, if an infant does not get consistent, safe, stable, and nurturing care, the crucial capacity to form and maintain healthy relationships won't develop. And depending upon a host of other developmental experiences, a range of problems with intimacy, social skills, and interpersonal behavior can develop.

*Oprah*: I know you've worked with people who never developed the ability to empathize.

*Dr. Perry*: I remember sitting in prison interviewing a woman who had murdered a young mother so she could take this mother's infant and raise it as her own. As I reviewed her records and talked with her, her disconnection was painfully clear.

But when you learn "what happened to her," it made sense. She herself had been abandoned when she was six days old. She then spent a few months in shelter care—where she had multiple caregivers—before entering the foster-care system. So from birth, she had no relational permanence whatsoever. She didn't belong to anyone; she didn't belong anywhere. By the time she was sixteen, she had lived in seven states, in twelve cities, at twenty-six different addresses. She never went to the same school for two years in a row. The longest she lived in any single place was eight months. She had no connection to family, to community, to place.

This woman was remorseless, expressing no real feeling for the mother she killed or the infant she took. As we talked, she felt empty and cold. She was lacking in empathy. But as we discussed in Chapter 3, you can't give what you don't get. If no one ever spoke to you, you can't speak; if you have never been loved, you can't be loving.

*Oprah*: But aside from extreme cases like hers, you've said there has been a shift in our collective ability be empathetic—to feel one another's pain.

*Dr. Perry*: Exactly. I'm talking about undeveloped or immature empathy. When young children hear fewer words, they can still learn to speak—they'll just be less fluent. In the same way, when children have fewer relational interactions, they'll still develop social capabilities—they'll just be less mature, more self-centered, more self-absorbed. This is what several studies are showing. There has been a significant drift in measures of empathy: The typical college-age adult is 30 percent "less empathic" and more self-absorbed than twenty years ago. One study documented a 40 percent increase in psychopathology in American college students over the last thirty years; the authors suggest that this is related to "cultural shifts towards extrinsic goals such as materialism and status and away from intrinsic goals, such as community, meaning in life, and affiliation." This is not to say that young people are bad or worse, but it's a clear example of how our life experiences shape us; what happens to you matters, and we all reflect to some degree the relational attributes of our family, community, and culture.

When I think about the changes in our family structure and our culture, I often think of the Barry Levinson film *Avalon*. The opening scene is a large multigenerational family gathering at Thanksgiving. The apartment is relatively small, but all the generations are there in their loving noisy chaos. Cut to the final scene, on a later Thanksgiving: After "making it" and moving to the suburbs, a nuclear family— once part of the big family—is sitting in parallel, not talking, eating frozen dinners on tray tables, and watching TV.

Our society's transgenerational social fabric is fraying. We're disconnecting. I think that's making us more vulnerable to adversity, and I think it's a significant factor in the increases in anxiety, suicide, and depression we are seeing currently, even before the COVID-19 pandemic.

*Oprah*: You think that's about disconnection.

*Dr. Perry*: Yes. Disconnection and loneliness in our society are playing a major role in the increased anxiety, sleep problems, substance use, and depression we're seeing.

A recent study by a team at Harvard found that of all the factors involved in depression, the most powerful were related to connectedness: "The protective effects of social connection were present even for individuals who were at higher risk for depression as a result of genetic vulnerability or early life trauma." Certainly, our work supports that observation. One of our major findings is that in determining someone's current mental health, the history of their childhood relational health—their connectedness—is as important as, if not more important than, their history of adversity. And for children and youth experiencing trauma, the best predictor of their current mental health functioning is their current connectedness.

I'm reminded of the Māori elders and their belief that trauma, anxiety, depression, and substance abuse are "all the same thing"—and all related to our connectedness, our sense of belonging.

Oprah: I agree. I have mentioned that one profound thing I realized, after listening to thousands of people share their story, is that all pain is the same—we just choose different ways to express it. And beyond that, I believe we are all here to learn from one another's pain. So the loss of community and the social isolation we all feel is a source of great collective pain.

Dr. Perry: Disconnection is disease. I think the Māori elders were right, and that there is some correlation between rising suicide rates and the increased fraying of our social fabric.

We are now raising our children and youth in environments that are both relationally impoverished and sensory overloading from the proliferation of screen-based technologies.

Oprah: We're all too attached to our phones. No one even makes eye contact.

Dr. Perry: Right. There's more texting, tweeting, and posting, but less actual conversation.

I believe we don't have enough quiet conversational moments listening to a friend with no other distractions. That kind of interaction leads to a completely different quality of human connection. A different depth. I think we crave that, and many of us turn to social media to find it, but ultimately those interactions don't satisfy the craving.

Meanwhile, rates of suicide, anxiety, and depression are rising in our youth. Our culture is so "advanced," and we have such wealth, creativity, and productivity—yet the disparities and inequities in all of our systems continue to marginalize, fragment, and undermine community and cultural cohesion.

We may have a pretty good public-education system, we may have amazing technologies, but we're still not meeting the fundamental relational needs of our children or ourselves. So many people feel empty and are seeking connection, and often seeking it in really unhealthy ways.

*Oprah*: And it happens at all socioeconomic levels. Wealth doesn't seem to stop anyone from having anxiety or depression.

*Dr. Perry*: True. But being on the bottom of any power differential makes life a lot harder. If you don't belong to the "in" group, your marginalization can contribute to feelings of not belonging.

As we talked about earlier, the brain is continually scanning the social environment for signals that tell you if you do or don't belong. When a person gets the signals—many of which are subconscious— that they belong, their stress-response systems quiet down, telling them they're safe. They feel regulated and rewarded. But when they get cues that they don't belong, their stress-response systems are activated. And "don't-belong" cues are our default response to anyone we don't know, especially if they don't have the attributes of our familiar group. We view this person as a potential threat.

*Oprah*: As the "other."

*Dr. Perry*: That's right. Now think about the implications of that for our modern world. As we mentioned, if you live in an urban area, you may see hundreds of "new" people every day, and your brain has to continually monitor these hundreds of people. *Friend or foe?* *Help me or hurt me?* It is taxing. It consumes emotional bandwidth. Often people living in urban settings learn to completely ignore and disengage with others. They may walk past you without any acknowledgement. The interaction makes you feel invisible, but for them it might just be a form of self-preservation.

Many people have had the experience of feeling "exhausted" after a day of travel, even if all they did was stand in a few lines and sit on a plane. This happens because your brain was continuously monitoring thousands of new stimuli. Remember: Activating your stress-response systems, even at a moderate level, for long periods of time is physically and emotionally exhausting.

So, part of the increase in anxiety in our modern world comes down to the constant bombardment of novelty—especially social novelty—and the absence of counterbalancing relational connection.

*Oprah*: So as our world expands and we encounter more and more people, the brain becomes overwhelmed.

*Dr. Perry*: Yes, and as a result, it will start to use shortcuts to manage all of these new people. Your brain can manage only a limited number of fully reciprocal relationships. Interestingly, in light of what we've been talking about, this number is about eighty to one hundred people—the size of a large hunter-gatherer band.

*Oprah*: It takes a lot of energy and time to get to know someone new, and there is only so much space in our brains. Maybe this is why moving is so hard.

*Dr. Perry*: Right. When you're new to a community, having moved away from what's familiar, your brain is going to be continually trying to manage all the novelty. And that's very hard to do without any real relational anchors in the new environment. The relationships will grow, but it takes time. This is why people are most vulnerable in the first six months after major transitions—after leaving the safe, stable, and known behind to start building a new set of connections.

Think of the girls at your school. They are incredible young women, but they've been taken out of their social context and put into a completely new environment. Until they can rebuild that connectedness, there's a vulnerability.

*Oprah*: That's why I try to find them host families, so they always have a place to go. A safe space.

*Dr. Perry*: That's a really smart thing to do, because connectedness is what helps us manage transitions and regulate in the face of a nonstop bombardment of novelty.

*Oprah*: And now, without community, what do people do? They look to their devices. There's nothing objectively wrong with it, but in the end it's a hollow connection.

*Dr. Perry*: I sometimes see an almost frenetic attempt to be connected by getting more "friends" or "followers" or "likes." There is such a powerful pull to belong, to make your clan, but as you say, social media connections are often hollow.

*Oprah*: Because it's not the "friends" or "followers" who stay by your side when you're sick or when you get divorced or just feel lonely. They're not sitting at the table with their neighbors—or even, in many cases, with their families.

I'm thinking back to what you said earlier—that disconnection is disease. Could isolation be categorized as a new form of trauma?

*Dr. Perry:* I do think that in some situations, isolation and loneliness can create a sensitization of the stress-response systems. So in that way they can be traumatic. For example, putting someone in solitary confinement. The timing of the isolation also makes a difference—think of the woman I met with in prison who'd been abandoned as a newborn.

I think it would certainly be reasonable to consider relational poverty—lack of connectedness—as an adversity. Poverty of relationship can disrupt normal development, influence how the brain works, put you at risk for physical and mental health problems. It's absolutely not good for you.

*Oprah:* Especially for children.

*Dr. Perry:* Yes. We all want to be part of a group, yet so many children are marginalized, excluded, or bullied. This can be devastating. Being left out can have a deep and enduring impact.

In many ways, the result of our society's poverty of relationships is a form of social and emotional starvation. Our children are starving.

*Oprah:* I think that's a difficult concept for most people to get, because children in our modern culture seem to have everything. What do you mean when you say they're starving?

*Dr. Perry:* Well, there are different forms of nourishment. One of the things we don't appreciate in Western cultures is how powerful and important touch is to our physical and emotional growth.

*Oprah:* Interesting.

*Dr. Perry:* Touch is as essential for healthy physical and emotional development as calories and vitamins. If infants aren't held or rocked—

if they don't experience the loving warmth of a caregiver's touch—they won't grow. In fact, they can die.

*Oprah*: Literally die?

*Dr. Perry*: Absolutely. And many people in our society, including children and youth, are touch-starved. Healthy touch is not well understood. We actually have schools where tiny toddlers whose impulse is to run up and hug a classmate or teacher are told not to touch; in return, the teachers and other caregivers are not allowed to touch the children. But it's simply unhealthy for a three- or four-year-old child to go eight hours without touching or hugging or playfully wrestling with another person.

*Oprah*: That's one of the things that so disturbed me when I heard about parents being separated from their children at the Mexico-U.S. border. Colleen Kraft, the former head of the American Academy of Pediatrics, said what struck her was that the caretakers weren't allowed to touch the toddlers. The babies are screaming and crying, and the caretakers have been told that they're not allowed to touch them. They just kept giving them toys and giving them toys and giving them toys. I *know* there is a way to allow healthy touch while protecting children from unwanted touch.

*Dr. Perry*: This is a classic example of making policy recommendations with good intentions but minimal understanding of the developmental needs of children. The intent is to help children by minimizing the potential for inappropriate touch or abuse, and at the same time protect staff from any false allegations. But rather than thinking through reasonable options to ensure healthy touch in a well-monitored setting, blanket "no touch" rules are applied.

This is a common thread in our culture: We're reactive; we prioritize convenient, short-term solutions; we're risk-averse; and we use material things rather than relationships as rewards. *Here, have a toy. Be good and we will give you a thing.* Giving toys instead of calming touch is an outrageously misguided practice. It's the result of developmentally ignorant, trauma-uninformed policies—and another example of the need to change our systems.

*Oprah*: When I heard that, it made me cry. We really do need to do better. We know better. We know that human contact is healthy. We know that too much time in front of a screen cannot replace a friend, teacher, coach, or parent.

*Dr. Perry*: Again, the speed with which we're inventing our world is outpacing our ability to understand the impact of our inventions. Television, video games, phones, computers—these are all pretty new. And we don't quite know the full impact of these devices on the developing brain, on how our children will think and process experience. But we are beginning to understand the disruptive impact that eleven hours in front of a screen can have on social development. We have all seen the disruptive effect of text messages or phone calls during a family dinner or a conversation with friends. And the distracting impact of surfing the internet during a lecture in school or a meeting at work.

*Oprah*: I've heard you use the phrase "techno-hygiene." I love that. Will you explain what it means?

*Dr. Perry*: Basically, I believe we need to develop social-practice "rules" about when and how to use our new technologies. We have always invented new rules as we've created new technologies.

Take current hygiene practices as an example. In the history of medicine, one of the most important advances was recognizing the relationships among disease, microbes, and sewage. It seems unbelievable to us now, but surgeons used to go into surgery without washing their hands; people went to the bathroom wherever they wanted, and communities dumped sewage into drinking-water sources. But as we learned about bacteria, infection, and disease, we realized we needed to manage things better. A host of hygiene protocols developed. We socialize children to go to the bathroom in the bathroom. We wash our hands after using the toilet. We keep our sewage away from our drinking water.

I think we need the same sort of universal "rules" for the standard use of our technologies. No-phone zones and no-phone times, proper "dosing" and spacing of screen time, and so forth. We know, for example, that nonstop screen time for a young child is not optimal for healthy development of language skills, attention, or concentration, so age and time limit recommendations have been made by the American Academy of Pediatrics. And as we learn more, we can develop and modify some of these "hygiene" recommendations.

*Oprah*: Isn't it true that children who are under the age of two or three should not even be looking at a tablet or screen because it's bad for the development of the brain?

*Dr. Perry*: It's probably not optimal.

*Oprah*: Why is that?

*Dr. Perry*: Our brain is organized in a way that makes us visually biased; though we have multiple senses, vision tends to be the dominant one. Images can evoke powerful responses because our brain has a preference for colorful and moving visual content. When you combine those two things on a screen, the viewer's attention is captured.

That's not necessarily bad—until it becomes so pleasing and engaging to the brain that we begin to prefer it to other less-stimulating, less-busy sensory input. An infant or toddler consumed by a screen is missing out on other critical forms of learning about the world. They should be exploring what things feel like, smell like, taste like. They should be making sense of their world using all their sensory tools.

You know how babies or toddlers are always putting things in their mouth? They're trying to see what a purple flower tastes like. They are making sense of the world. But if 75 percent of your day is spent staring at a screen, not touching, feeling, moving, or interacting with other human beings, you're essentially underdeveloping key parts of the brain that are rapidly organizing at that time of life.

The best way to teach a child language isn't to put them in front of a screen, it's to talk with them. When you actually look at children's language acquisition, you see that fluency is related to the number of words spoken in a back-and-forth, interactive, conversational way. Not the number of words heard on a device.

*Oprah*: And we want children to make real-life connections with other children and adults. As you said, the empathy systems in the brain develop when there are many opportunities for stimulation.

*Dr. Perry*: So, ideally, if a child is growing up in a relationally "wealthy" home, with lots of opportunities for safe, stable, and nurturing interactions, they will be building their connectedness and resilience. This insight was a core understanding of all the traditional child-rearing and healing practices I learned about from Indigenous elders.

Their understanding of the primacy of human connectedness reflects a wisdom lost in our current world. How ironic that the cultures our modern world has marginalized are the very cultures with the wisdom to heal our modern woes.

# CHAPTER 10

——

# WHAT
# WE NEED
# NOW

Years ago, I played the character of Sethe in the film version of Toni Morrison's searing novel Beloved.

Sethe was a former slave, haunted by the horrific death of her daughter, Beloved. In the film, Beloved returns to Sethe, reincarnated as a disabled child Sethe takes into her home. For the rest of her life, Sethe does penance to Beloved as their relationship becomes more and more debilitating and intertwined.

One day we were shooting a scene where Sethe was supposed to tuck Beloved into bed. The only instruction I got from the director, Jonathan Demme, was, "Okay, tuck her in."

And so I walked to each corner of the bed and folded the blanket down perfectly and tucked it under the mattress.

"Cut," Jonathan yelled from behind the camera. "Oprah, you're not tucking her in."

And so I repeated the process more purposefully, tucking each corner of the blanket under the mattress.

"Cut!" Jonathan walked over to me. "What are you doing?"

"I'm tucking her in." I could feel a mix of fear and embarrassment rising inside me, but I didn't know why.

"You're making the bed," he said. "Not tucking in your daughter for bed."

In that moment, something clicked. Deeply. I stared at Jonathan. "I don't know what 'tucking in' means," I said quietly. "I don't know how to do that."

Finally we both understood what was happening. Jonathan gently taught me how to circle my daughter with loving tucks of the blanket. As we moved around the bed together, I was hit by a flood of grief.

I don't recall ever being tucked in.

I never felt anyone place a blanket on me with that kind of loving intention.

That must be what a mother's love is.

*Years later, I was in the kitchen with my friend Urania, and her young daughter, Kylee. Urania asked Kylee if she'd like something to eat. "Yes, please," Kylee said.*

*Urania went to the refrigerator and took out some strawberries. She washed them, took a knife, and began slicing. I could see she'd done this many times before. As the knife moved around a berry, the shape of a delicate rose began to emerge. "A strawberry rose!" I marveled. Urania carefully placed the beautiful berries on a plate and handed them to her daughter. Watching, my eyes filled with tears. The tenderness with which she did it seared my soul.*

*Again, I said to myself, "That must be what a mother's love is."*

*My mother and I had a complicated relationship. As I mentioned earlier, I spent my early childhood—my first six years—living with my grandmother. I have no memory of my mother during that period.*

*When my grandmother became sick, I was suddenly moved to Milwaukee to live with my mother. This was not a joyful maternal-child reunion. I could feel I was not welcome.*

*The night I arrived in Milwaukee, the woman my mother was boarding with, Ms. Miller, took one look at me and said, "She'll have to sleep on the porch." Ms. Miller was light-skinned. She could almost pass for white, and she was not going to have this "nappy-headed dark child," as she said, stay in the house.*

*My mother said, "All right."*

*I had never slept anywhere but in my grandmother's bed. On the enclosed porch, I could hear noise from the street. As I watched my mother close the house door to go to the bed where I'd thought I'd sleep, I was consumed with a terrified sense of loneliness that brought me to tears. I imagined a robber snatching me from the porch or someone breaking through the windows and choking me. That first night, I got on my knees and prayed to God to send angels to protect me.*

*When I woke in the morning, the terror was gone, but the sense of being unsafe while sleeping would remain for much of my life. A knowing had filled my soul. At six years old, I felt I was alone and no one but God was going to watch out for me.*

*My pain and the resolve that followed it became a cycle that would repeat itself many times. I believe it is, in a profound way, the very through line of my life. The struggles I endured as a child are what allowed me to recognize and care about pain in others. The validation I longed for as a child is what I see other people longing for just as intensely. Thousands of people had the courage to share their stories with me because their story was my story. Their pain was my pain. Because all pain is the same.*

—Oprah

*Oprah*: There are so many beautiful stories of people who say they were able to "break the cycle" of abuse or trauma in their family. Is it possible to completely prevent passing on the negative or toxic effects of such experiences?

*Dr. Perry*: It's important to clarify that most people who are abused don't go on to abuse others in the same way. On the other hand, it is becoming clear that it's the very rare person who has been abused who doesn't have some form of adaptation that impacts how they deal with people. It doesn't have to be a "pathology," but it can influence the ways in which you form and maintain relationships.

This goes back to our earlier talk about why some people seem to seek abusive relationships. Our brain, our mind, pulls us toward familiar patterns—even when those patterns are negative. People end up repeating previous maladaptive patterns and often don't recognize it. A lot of times, the people around us will see it more clearly than we do.

*Oprah*: Yes, and so often real change can't happen until you do see it for yourself. I knew very early on in my childhood that if I was going to make it, I was going to have to do it on my own. There was no scaffolding, as you call it, built for me. But over the years, there were some very special teachers who took the time to nurture the potential they recognized in me. And that's what you are saying. It really can be just a handful of people seeing you through a new lens and taking time to help. My teachers didn't have a trauma-informed education. Now that some people have, and now that your groundbreaking work is out in the world making ripple effects, are you hopeful that more people can heal?

*Dr. Perry*: I'm more hopeful than I was twenty years ago. I've spent most of my career trying to better understand and help children, youth, and adults after trauma. For us, a major advancement came when we could finally translate some of the complex neuroscience into useful models for clinical work.

The Neurosequential Model allows us to create a version of how the individual's brain appears to be organized; it is basically like an inspection of a house. By asking about the "history" of the house's construction—the "what happened to you?"—we are able to home in on the most likely problems. What would predictably happen if you didn't let the cement of the foundation set, or didn't properly route the plumbing up to the second floor?

Once we know the source of the problem, we can better understand how to fix it. In a sequence that replicates the original construction of the house—the brain—we put in place a "rebuilding/renovation" plan. With the problem areas in mind, we can provide experiences—both educational and therapeutic—that jump-start and reorganize the systems that were impacted by neglect, adversity, and trauma. We have a better idea about how to select and sequence therapeutic experiences—a better grasp of what we can do to help, and when.

We have a lot more to learn, but we're pretty optimistic. Hundreds of thousands of children, youth, and adults from over twenty-six countries have benefited from clinical and educational services that use this neurodevelopmental, trauma-aware lens.

Think back to Mike Roseman. When we finally started the "bottom-up" approach that helped regulate his trauma-sensitized CRNs, that was a beta version of the Neurosequential Model approach—addressing the brain's problems in the proper sequence and focusing on the lower networks before moving on to issues in the higher regions.

*Oprah*: Regulate, relate, then reason, as you say.

*Dr. Perry*: Let me give you one additional, even more detailed example of how this works. About twenty years ago we were asked to see Susan, a seven-year-old girl who'd been adopted at age two; her behaviors were overwhelming her parents, teachers, and therapists.

At age two, when she was adopted, Susan was nonverbal and had sleep problems, prolonged "temper tantrums," staring spells, and self-mutilation behaviors like scratching her face and picking at her skin until it bled. As she got older, physical and occupational therapists, tutors, live-in mental health specialists, in-school aides, developmental pediatricians, psychologists, and psychiatrists were involved in her care. She'd been through five years of shifting diagnostic labels and treatments, with minimal progress.

Early in her life, Susan had profound adversity and minimal relational connection. The "foundation" of her house was very likely weak and fragile. She was born to a single mother who struggled with mental health problems; the mother had been removed from her own parents when she was four and spent her entire childhood and youth in a series of foster homes. At eighteen, she aged out of the system and was on her own. She immediately became pregnant but was unable to care for Susan. The child welfare system removed Susan at four months of age and ultimately terminated parental rights. Susan became a ward of the state. This form of transgenerational trauma is not uncommon with so many of the children in our child-protective systems.

When Susan was removed from her mother, she entered shelter care for two months. Then she was in a succession of three foster homes before she was finally adopted. One can only imagine her "worldview" about the safety and trustworthiness of adults. The process of building her house was continually interrupted; the wiring, plumbing, and framing were all impacted by a two-year span of unpredictable, uncontrollable, and extreme activation of her stress-response systems. It was no surprise that she had classic symptoms of a sensitized dissociative system. Her self-mutilation, as we have talked about before, was an attempt to regulate herself.

In the face of unavoidable pain and distress, she dissociated—hence her staring spells. And the arousal component of her stress response was also sensitized (see Figure 5): Her temper tantrums were the toddler's equivalent of the flight-or-fight response. This was a terrified, confused, undeveloped child.

Now, part of the problem was that the educational and mental-health systems—not to mention her parents—viewed Susan as a seven-year-old child. But while she was chronologically seven, she wasn't developmentally seven. She had the social skills of an infant, the regulatory skills of a two-year-old, the cognitive skills of a three-year-old. Parents, teachers, and therapists kept trying to reason with her. They explained the rules and tried to explore "why" she did all these "naughty" things. They were doing the best they could; they did not understand state-dependent functioning or the developmental challenges that were predictable considering Susan's history.

Our Neurosequential Model allowed us to create a blueprint for therapeutics that started with the "foundation"—the bottom parts of Susan's brain. She had significant sensory-integration issues—she couldn't stand being touched; when more than one person was talking in a room she was overwhelmed; she wouldn't tolerate certain fabrics on her skin; she was always burying herself beneath piles of pillows and blankets and more—so we started by creating a set of predictable and patterned somatosensory experiences: weighted blankets, gradually introduced therapeutic massage, an enriched "sensory diet" provided by a trauma-aware occupational therapist. We didn't focus on Susan's problems with peers, her inability to pay attention in class, her depressive symptoms, her explosive outbursts, or even her speech problems. We were going in sequence. We started with the lower systems, knowing we'd get to the other problems later in the treatment process.

A key part of a neurosequential approach is to help parents, teachers, and clinicians know the "stage" and watch the "state." Meaning we want to help them learn what the child's actual developmental capabilities are—their actual stage, as opposed to their age. And we want to help them become aware of the child's state-dependence; we encourage them to ask themselves, "Is this child in a state where they can effectively 'hear' what I'm trying to say or teach?"

It is amazing how often we ignore this. As we have discussed, if the child is too dysregulated, they will not be open to any new learning or experience. And if you continue to expect the child to pay attention, focus, and learn, you will be eroding the child's sense of safety with you. You will be damaging the empathic bond between the two of you—the very thing on which all chance of change depends. So back away from "teaching," "coaching," and "reasoning" when the child's state is such that they cannot learn. Focus on being present and regulate yourself when you start to feel frustrated, disrespected, or angry because they have not listened to you. If you step away and calm down, you will have access to your cortex to then remember ways to help regulate the child. Your relationship lives to teach another day.

Our work with Susan continued for four years. She made slow but steady progress. The primary therapeutic techniques evolved—from somatosensory to rhythmic and regulatory (including working with a therapy dog) to relational, and finally to cognitive-dominant (like trauma-focused cognitive-behavioral therapy, or TF-CBT). The fascinating thing is that we ended up using many of the same therapeutic methods that had previously failed. There hadn't been anything inherently "wrong" with the prior methods—they were simply applied at a time when Susan couldn't benefit from them. Neurosequential. It's all about the sequence. The brain develops, processes incoming sensory input, and heals in sequence.

By the end of this therapeutic process, Susan was in a mainstream classroom and on grade level; she had a handful of friends; she had no more explosive or self-mutilation behaviors. She had transitioned to healthier, more socially acceptable forms of dissociative regulation—reading, art, and drama. She was developing her capacity to be kind and compassionate. Her parents were no longer exhausted and burned out.

*Oprah*: And the lesson is that no matter what has happened, you get a chance to rewrite the script.

*Dr. Perry*: Exactly. It really is never too late. Healing is possible. The key is knowing where to start the process. And matching the developmental needs of the person.

*Oprah*: I remember talking to Belinda Pittman-McGee, who runs the Nia Imani center, in Milwaukee, a long-term transitional housing facility for homeless young women who are pregnant or have young children. Belinda said that women often come to the center with behavioral disorders like a quick temper or the inability to hold a job—the kinds of things that can come from being raised in a traumatic environment. When she starts teaching them about trauma, she says they begin to understand that their struggles with emotions and acting out are connected to "what happened to them." That realization in itself can be life-changing when you've labeled yourself as bad or stupid and believed that was your fate.

*Dr. Perry*: I can't tell you how many people feel incredibly relieved when they get an explanation of how their brain is working, and why. We don't give them a psychiatric label. We're just saying this is the way you're organized and it's absolutely predictable based upon *what happened to you*. Then we help them understand that the brain is malleable, "plastic," changeable. And together we come up with a plan that will help change some of the systems that appear to be causing them problems.

*Oprah*: It's the recognition that *What I've* been through *has caused me to have these kinds of feelings. And I'm not the only one. And it makes sense.* It makes sense that if you're an overworked mother of three or four with a history of trauma, you'll have trouble coping while trying to carry your burdens all by yourself. Your health is being compromised in ways you don't even recognize.

And then to realize that the reason you feel so overwhelmed is that you haven't found a good way to regulate yourself. This is why giving back to yourself is so important. If you aren't regulated yourself, how can you parent or work effectively?

*Dr. Perry*: That is such an important point. We are often asked to help children and youth who have been maltreated or traumatized, or consult for a community following a traumatic event. And when I tell people that I'll actually need to work with the adults, too, they're confused. But if the adults who live with, teach, and treat these children are not regulated, they will not be able to be fully present in a compassionate, regulated way. It is those fully present moments that are regulating, rewarding, and healing for the children. If we help the children but don't meet the needs of the adults, our work will have little impact. This is one of the most important principles of any trauma-informed approach: You have to help the frontline adults who will be working with the children and youth.

This shift in focus is challenging for some of our systems. In the child mental health system, for example, the "patient" is the child. The system's economic model typically doesn't include paying a clinician if they want to give time to the child's teacher, coach, or even parents. This is short-sighted. We know that a dysregulated adult cannot regulate a dysregulated child. An exhausted, frustrated, dysregulated adult can't regulate anybody.

As you point out, if you don't give back to yourself, you simply will not be effective as a teacher, a leader, a supervisor, a parent, a coach, anything. Self-care is huge. Unfortunately, many people feel some guilt about taking care of themselves; they view self-care as selfish. It's not selfish—it is essential. Remember, the major tool you have in helping others change—whether you are a parent, teacher, coach, therapist, or friend—is *you*. Relationships are the currency of change.

*Oprah*: We have to take care of ourselves so we can *bring* ourselves. This is especially important considering that so many of us are walking around with trauma or adversity in our own pasts. I wouldn't be who I am without my trauma. So I own it. I claim it. And, by doing that, I believe I have found a way to use it in service to others. Empathy, compassion, and forgiveness. These are all part of the practice that moves me forward in every decision or encounter I experience.

*Dr. Perry*: Yes, that brings us back to post-traumatic wisdom. When you've lived through adversity, you can come to a point in your life where you can look back, reflect, learn, and grow from the experience. I believe it's hard to understand humankind unless you know a little bit about adversity. Adversity, challenges, disappointment, loss, trauma—all can contribute to the capacity to be broadly empathic, to become wise. Trauma and adversity, in a way, are gifts. What we do with these gifts will differ from person to person.

*Oprah*: It's so interesting to hear you say that. When I was growing up, I wanted to live like *Leave It to Beaver*. That was my idea of what a family should be—milk and cookies at home, Mom and Dad together, the whole thing. But I wouldn't have become the evolved human being that I'm still in the process of becoming if I'd had everything at my disposal or had everything I wanted at exactly the moment I thought I wanted it.

*Dr. Perry*: I feel the same way. It is true, though, that the cost of wisdom can be very high. And for many people, the pain never goes away. The wise learn how to carry their burden with grace, often to protect others from the emotional intensity of their pain.

*Oprah*: This makes me think of Anthony Ray Hinton, the man who served thirty years on death row for a murder he didn't commit. For the first three years of his sentence, he did not speak at all. He was so depressed and desolate, he said he felt like God took away his voice. The thing that allowed him to survive was his ability to dissociate. He turned to his imagination and gave himself all kinds of experiences. He played in Wimbledon and won five times. He played in the NBA, he met the Queen of England, he was married to Halle Berry—and he did it all in his mind.

*Dr. Perry*: He was able to use his dissociative superpower to protect himself from the uncontrollable, unavoidable pain of his imprisonment.

*Oprah*: And then he found a way to turn it to good—the wisdom and grace you're talking about. After he started connecting with the other inmates on death row, he convinced the warden to let them start a book club. He thought they didn't know how to travel in their minds the way he did, but books could let them do that. He wanted them to have a way to start to heal, as he had started to heal.

You know, throughout all our many conversations, I keep going back to a show I did with Iyanla Vanzant years ago. She said that until you heal the wounds of your past, you will continue to bleed. The wounds will bleed through and stain your life, through alcohol, through drugs, through sex, through overworking. You have to have the courage to pull out the wound and begin to heal yourself.

This is the lesson I hope everyone carries with them from our conversation, too. We must understand and heal the wounds of the past before we can move forward.

*Dr. Perry*: I can't help thinking the same is true for a society, not just an individual. How can our society move toward a more humane, socially just, creative, and productive future without confronting our collective historical trauma? Both trauma experienced and trauma inflicted. If we truly want to understand ourselves, we need to understand our history—our true history. Because the emotional residue of our past follows us.

*Oprah*: But that can't happen until there is a tipping point of awareness—of what we have done to ourselves as human beings, of what the true human condition is, of what trauma has done to us. That's when there will be a realization that we need to do something different.

*Dr. Perry*: The core elements are awareness coupled with connectedness. Together, these can create a trauma-informed community.

*Oprah*: I think that's what the world truly needs more of right now. When you're able to really see another person, that's true compassion, and extending yourself in compassion to another human being changes the nature of our relationships, our communities, and our world. The acknowledgment of one human being by another is what bonds us. Asking "What happened to you?" expands the human connection.

*Dr. Perry*: It is easy to be discouraged and overwhelmed by the many problems in our society, to be demoralized by the inequities, adversities, and trauma that are all too pervasive in our world. But if you study history, you will recognize that the overall trajectory for humankind is positive. Our world is filled with so many kind, capable, and creative people. We are a curious species. We will continue to discover, invent, and learn. We can make our world a safer, more just, and humane place for all.

# EPILOGUE

The young man was standing waist-deep in the pool, leading an aqua-fitness class for the elderly. He was wearing a blue T-shirt with the logo of the retirement home, a lanyard with a whistle, and a large name tag. I couldn't read the name, but I knew it: Jesse, the young man from Chapter 3. The last time I'd seen him, ten years earlier, he was unconscious in a hospital bed.

I watched through a window as Jesse enthusiastically led eight members of the retirement community through their paces. He moved from person to person smiling, correcting their stances, gently helping one woman with her shoulder. It was clear that they liked him and he liked them. He was having fun; they were having fun. He belonged.

When I originally evaluated Jesse, it was a consultation for a clinical team in another state. After the initial in-person consultation, which took place while Jesse was still in a coma, I continued to track his progress and consult to his team from a distance. After a month or so, Jesse "woke up." Initially he had signs of severe brain damage, but slowly, all of his functioning returned, with the exception of some aspects of his long-term memory, especially "narrative" memory. His "autobiographical" memory of life before the coma was in disorganized shards. When asked about people, places, and events, he simply couldn't remember. The neurology team thought this was related to his brain injury. Having seen multiple cases of amnesia following trauma, I wasn't so sure. My recommendation was to let that go for the time being. Let's get him back to walking, talking, moving, socializing. We can track his memory, focus on short-term memory skills. Most important, let's get him into a safe, stable, and nurturing placement for the first time in his life.

Initially, Jesse needed a special-needs placement due to his rehabilitation plan. The social worker on the team—who was a lot smarter than I—suggested that we place him in a local retirement community that had a continuum of living situations, from independent living condominiums to "dorm-like" single rooms to more traditional high-needs rehab beds. Several of the community's senior staff members were given on-site housing as part of their compensation; the social worker's partner was one of these staff members. The two of them lived together "on campus" at the retirement community, and they agreed to "foster" Jesse. It was a true community—multiple buildings, a garden, a gym with a pool and exercise rooms, a library, hairdresser, several dining rooms, and a coffee shop. The placement was genius.

Jesse moved in and immediately was embraced by the staff and residents. Though in the beginning he was "home-schooled," within a year he was able to walk down the street to the public school. He was able to manage the academic content; he had no behavioral problems at home or school. But while he made a few friends, he was never very close to or comfortable with his peers—he was liked by all, but not really embraced by any. His best relationships were with his foster parents and the elderly residents. He started working as a transportation aide, helping residents move throughout the complex and get to their various appointments in the community. He learned to drive. At eighteen, he was allowed to move into one of the independent-living placements right next to his foster parents. He graduated from high school. Now, at twenty-three, he was legally independent but connected to his foster parents and considered a part of their family. He was in community college part-time, focusing on physical education classes with aspirations of becoming a physical therapist. At the retirement community he had advanced to the role of assistant recreation director, with part of his compensation being his housing and board. He had found his safe, stable, and nurturing home. Thousands upon thousands of unstructured therapeutic moments in his community had helped him heal.

From time to time I would hear from my colleagues and get an update. I still wondered about Jesse's memory. He'd had a horrific childhood—abuse in many forms along with relational betrayal, neglect, unspeakable degradation. Yet as he recovered from his head *injury, he was not impulsive, aggressive, inattentive, or hostile. Although he had physiological reactivity to certain evocative cues, he did not have PTSD or other readily observable trauma-related symptoms. His emotional and behavioral functioning never caused the adult world—or him—to reach out for mental health help.*

*Dr. Anderson was his neurologist and had been working with Jesse all these years. Knowing that I was coming to town, I'd asked him how Jesse was doing. He suggested I see for myself and asked Jesse if he'd be willing to have lunch with me.*

*"You will not remember this, Jesse," I said when we met, "but I was one of the doctors working with Dr. Anderson back when you had your brain injury. Thanks for agreeing to see me."*

*He smiled and put his hand out. "Well, thank you for helping me back then."*

*We walked to the cafeteria-style dining room, stood in line to select our lunch, and sat down to talk. Small talk. He asked about Texas; I asked about his school. We went back and forth like that until he asked, politely, "Did you come here to analyze me?"*

*I joked back, "No. You'd have to pay me for that."*

*He smiled. We looked at each other, each of us fully present in a silent, connected moment.*

*"I do wonder about your memory, though."*

*A slow sadness came over his face. He gazed down into a space filled with some painful memory. I let the sounds of the cafeteria wash over the moment.*

*An elderly woman came over and kissed Jesse on the forehead. "Thank you for the flowers," she said. "They made my day."*

*The gesture broke his gaze, and the animated, smiling Jesse emerged. "I knew you would like them. Let's go out to the garden this afternoon and get some more."*

*As she walked away, Jesse seemed embarrassed. Not by their interaction, but by the earlier moment of sadness. "When you first were recovering from your head injury, Dr. Anderson said you had no memory of your childhood," I offered.*

*Jesse shrugged. "I really don't like to think about all that."*

*"We don't have to talk about any of this if you don't want to, Jesse."*

*"It's okay. I just don't like to think about it, and I don't like to upset anyone."*

*"I understand. You probably know that I work with many people—children and adults—who have had terrible life experiences. And each one of them has helped me better understand how to help others. So when you are ready, I would love to learn from you." He studied me as I spoke. "You had a really hard start in life, Jesse. And now, here you are, after all you went through, going to school, you have a great job, lots of great relationships, and you seem pretty happy. I suspect you could teach me a lot."*

*"I do have trouble sleeping sometimes."*

*I nodded.*

*"But then I just get up and work out, go for a run. That really helps. And I get really nervous around too many people. Really just want to go back home whenever I'm out too much."*

*"But you're always around people here, Jesse."*

*"Yeah. That's true. I mean, I don't really like being around younger people, children. Too loud, too crazy."*

*In that moment, I realized that many of his evocative cues were from the catalog of sensory stimuli from children and childhood. Children's voices, smells, games, cartoons, foods, anything—his childhood was so permeated with threat that his brain, struggling to make sense of the world, associated almost everything in his small, abusive world with threat. But his new life, his "reset" redo life, was in a world of the elderly. The retirement home was filled with sensory experiences entirely different from those in a class full of children or a group home for youth. The type of movement, the speed of movement, the pitch of voices, the scents, images, schedules, music, television preferences—all were different. Relational interactions were different as well—more parallel and less evocative than those of his childhood. The placement had been even more genius than I'd realized. There were simply far fewer evocative cues to dysregulate Jesse in this setting. He was able to have more moderate, predictable, and controllable experiences here. He had more control over interactions; he pushed people in wheelchairs; they depended on him. Over time he was able to build a whole new catalog of "safe and familiar" that provided the foundation for his healing. And the thousands of positive, healing interactions over the ten years of this stable existence built him up.*

*"So, the memory loss. . . . ?" I asked.*

*He looked at me with the tiniest of bittersweet smiles. "I pretty much remember everything."*

*"Yeah, I figured. One of the things I've learned over the years is that what happened to you doesn't just go away. Those childhood experiences can impact you in many ways. And there are ways to help people heal. So if any of your memories ever bother you or you feel confused or upset, don't hesitate to reach out. There are ways to help make the trauma easier to carry." I gave him my card.*

*After lunch ended, a gaggle of elderly women swept him off to his next exercise session, a modified Zumba class. As he walked down the hall, he looked at my card in his hand, turned to wave, and danced away.*

*We talk a couple of times a year. Jesse's doing just fine. We're both still learning.*

—Dr. Perry

On November 22, 2018, my mother, Vernita Lee, passed away.

I was conflicted about our relationship up until the very end.

The truth is, it wasn't until I became successful that my mother started to show more interest in me. I wrestled with the question of how to take care of her. What did I owe the woman who gave me life? The Bible says, "Honor thy father and mother," but what did that actually mean?

I decided that one of the ways I could honor her would be to help care for her financially. I always made sure she had everything she needed in order to live a comfortable life, but there was never any real connection. I would say that the audience who watched me on television knew me better than my mother did.

When her health began to decline a few years ago, I knew I needed to prepare myself for her transition. Just a few days before Thanksgiving, my sister Patricia called to tell me she thought it was time. I flew to Milwaukee.

I sat with my mother for hours in a room she liked to keep at around eighty degrees. We watched Steve Harvey game shows and One Life to Live on a loop. I tried to think of something to say. At one point, I even picked up the manual left by the hospice care people. I read their advice—thinking the whole time how sad it was that I, Oprah Winfrey, who'd spoken to thousands of people one-on-one, should have to read a hospice manual to figure out what to say to my mother.

When it was finally time to leave, something told me it would be the last time I'd ever see her. But as I turned to go, the words still wouldn't come. All I could muster was, "Bye. . . . I'll be seeing you." And I left for, ironically, a speaking engagement.

On the flight home that night, the little voice in my head suddenly whispered what I knew in my heart to be true: "You're going to regret this. You haven't finished the work." In that moment, I felt like a hypocrite; if anyone else had been in my shoes, I'd have told them, "You need to go back and say the thing that needs to be said."

*I turned around and went back to Milwaukee.*

*Spent another day in that hot room, and still no words came.*

*That night I prayed for help. In the morning I meditated. As I prepared to head out the door, I picked up my phone and noticed the song that was playing—Mahalia Jackson singing "Precious Lord." If ever there was a sign, this was it. I have no idea how Mahalia Jackson appeared on my playlist. As I listened to the words—"Precious Lord, take my hand / Lead me on, let me stand / I am tired, I am weak, I am worn / Lead me on through the light. Take my hand"—I suddenly knew what to do.*

*When I walked into my mother's room, I asked if she wanted to hear the song. She nodded. And then I had another idea: I called my friend Wintley Phipps, a preacher and gospel artist, and asked him to sing "Precious Lord" to my dying mother. Over FaceTime, from his breakfast table, he sang the song a cappella and then prayed that our family would have "no fear, just peace."*

*I could see that my mother was moved. The song and the prayer had created a sort of opening—for both of us.*

*I began to talk to her, about her life, her dreams, and me.*

*Finally, the words were there.*

*I said, "It must have been hard for you. Not having an education, not having a skill, not knowing what the future held when you became pregnant. I'm sure a lot of people told you to get rid of that baby."*

*She nodded.*

*"But you didn't," I said. "And I want to thank you for keeping that baby." I paused. "I know that many times, you didn't know what to do. You did the best you knew how to do—and that's okay with me. That is okay with me. So you can leave now, knowing that it is well. It is well with my soul. It's been well for a long time."*

*It was a sacred, beautiful moment, one of the proudest of my life. As an adult I had learned to see my mother through a different lens— not as the mother who didn't care for me, protect me, love me, or* understand anything about me, but as a young girl, still just a child herself, scared, alone, and unequipped to be a loving parent.

I'd forgiven my mother years earlier for not being the mother I needed, but she didn't know that. And in our last moments together, I believe I was able to release her from the shame and the guilt of the past.

I came back and I finished the work that needed to be done.

Forgiveness is giving up the hope that the past could have been any different. But we cannot move forward if we're still holding on to the pain of that past. All of us who have been broken and scarred by trauma have the chance to turn those experiences into what Dr. Perry and I have been talking about: post-traumatic wisdom.

Forgive yourself, forgive them. Step out of your history and into the path of your future.

My friend, the poet Mark Nepo, says that the pain was necessary in order to know the truth.

But we don't have to keep the pain alive in order to keep the truth alive.

I made peace with my mother when I stopped comparing her to the mother I wished I had. When I stopped clinging to what should or could have been and turned to what was and what could be.

Because what I know for sure is that everything that has happened to you was also happening for you. And all that time, in all of those moments, you were building strength.

Strength times strength times strength equals power.

What happened to you can be your power.

—Oprah

# RESOURCES

Our hope is that this book has caused you to reflect on how you understand yourself and others, and that we have piqued your interest. The scope of trauma-related topics is wide, and the implications of developmental adversity are pervasive and profound. So, certainly we couldn't cover all of these in the finite pages of our book; if you want to learn more, here are some good places to start.

FOR MORE READING:

*The Boy Who Was Raised as a Dog: And Other Stories from
a Child Psychiatrist's Notebook*
Bruce D. Perry, M.D., Ph.D., and Maia Szalavitz
This book, originally published in 2006 and revised and updated in 2017, traces the evolution of Dr. Perry's work with children and youth impacted by neglect, trauma, and developmental adversity. It is an excellent complement to this book and provides a "deeper dive" into some of the core concepts discussed in *What Happened to You?*

*The Body Keeps the Score: Brain, Mind, and Body in the
Healing of Trauma*
Bessel van der Kolk, M.D.
Dr. van der Kolk is a pioneer and innovator in the field of trauma. This classic book, published in 2014, outlines the development of his research, clinical approach, and thinking about the complex effects of trauma on the brain, mind, and body.

*Born for Love: Why Empathy Is Essential—and Endangered*
Maia Szalavitz and Bruce D. Perry, M.D., Ph.D.

Published in 2010, this book uses stories and case examples to illustrate the crucial role that empathy—and love—plays in development and health. The authors emphasize the importance of being aware of the shifting of social connectedness in the modern world and address many of the topics related to "connectedness" discussed in *What Happened to You?*

*Together: The Healing Power of Human Connection in a*
*Sometimes Lonely World*
Vivek H. Murthy, M.D.
In this book, published in 2020, Dr. Vivek H. Murthy, the Surgeon General for Presidents Obama and Biden, addresses the importance of human connection and the impact of loneliness on our physical and emotional health. These messages echo many of the conversations in *What Happened to You?* and *Born for Love*, but his perspective as a physician leader examines these issues from a unique and important angle.

*The Deepest Well: Healing the Long-Term Effects of*
*Childhood Adversity*
Nadine Burke Harris, M.D.
This book, published in 2018, describes how Dr. Harris, the first Surgeon General of California, came to learn about the 1998 ACE studies and the correlations these studies documented between childhood trauma and risk for physical health problems. More important, she advocates for changes in health care that will help identify, prevent, and address the impact of adverse childhood experiences on health.

## TO LEARN MORE ABOUT:

### THE BRAIN AND NEUROSCIENCES:
*BrainFacts.Org:* This is the most reliable, accurate, and accessible resource for anyone interested in the brain. It is a public information

initiative that is a collaboration between the Society for Neuroscience, the Kavli Foundation, and the Gatsby Charitable Foundation. With materials for teachers, students, and professionals, this is a superb starting point for a deeper dive into the brain.

**PREVENTION OF ABUSE AND SUPPORTS FOR FAMILIES:**
*Prevent Child Abuse America (Preventchildabuse.org):* This is the nation's oldest and largest organization dedicated to prevention. This site is a great starting place to learn more about innovative, supportive programs for families proven to reduce abuse and neglect.

**ADVERSE CHILDHOOD EXPERIENCES (ACES):**
*Adverse Childhood Experiences section of the Violence Prevention Branch of the CDC (https://www.cdc.gov/violenceprevention/aces/index .html):* This site is a treasure trove of educational resources, research articles, and policy implications related to adverse childhood experiences. It is the most reliable resource for accurate information about ACEs.

**THE NEUROSEQUENTIAL MODEL AND THE WORK OF DR. PERRY:**
*The Neurosequential Network (Neurosequential.com):* This site outlines the research, clinical programs, and other educational activities of the Neurosequential Network (a community of practice spanning 28 countries and dozens of disciplines).

Visit *WhatHappenedtoYouBook.com* for a complete list of publications referenced in this book, and for more resources related to trauma, resilience, and healing.

## CREDITS AND ACKNOWLEDGMENTS

The authors are grateful to all of the children, youth, and adults who have shared their lives with us. Their stories are gifts of vulnerability and courage. Writing a book is a very collaborative effort. We would like to thank the many people from Harpo, Flatiron, Melcher Media, the Neurosequential Network, and others who gave their time, energy, and creativity to help with this book. We would like to give special thanks to Jenna Kostelnik Utley, Bryn Clark, and Lauren Nathan for leading this process. The Senior Leadership team of the Neurosequential Network—Jana Rosenfelt, Emily Perry, Diane Vines, Steve Graner, Erin Hambrick, and Kristie Brandt—deserve special recognition for the quality and evolution of much of Dr. Perry's work represented in this book.

This book was produced by

**MELCHER
MEDIA**

Founder and CEO: Charles Melcher
Vice President and COO: Bonnie Eldon
Editorial Director: Lauren Nathan
Production Director: Susan Lynch
Executive Editor: Chris Steighner
Senior Editor: Megan Worman
Senior Digital Producer: Shannon Fanuko
Editorial Assistant: Vanina Morrison

MELCHER MEDIA WOULD LIKE TO THANK
Chika Azuma, Luke Gernert, Carolyn Merriman, Cheryl Della Pietra, and Zoe Margolis.